Pharmaceutical Packaging and Single-Use Syringes

TECHNOLOGY AND TESTS

Dr. Abdrhman Mahmoud Gamil

Associate Professor of Pharmaceutics
Alneelain University, National University
Sudan

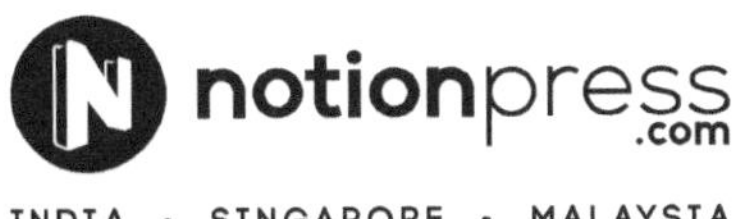

ISBN
Paperback 979-8-89724-287-0
Hardcase 979-8-89724-972-5

We are going to leave but traces will remain,
may Allah bless.

Dedication

To those who are striving to recover our homeland.

To those who had been killed or suffering from being displaced without any guilt they did.

To those who are suffering from hunger, diseases or obligated to leave their homes and belongings in order to survive.

To that group of lovers who struggle and work hard to fulfil their needs and keeping their lovers alive.

To those young men whom their educational pathway was disrupted and lost many valuable years of their lives due to the war and political instability.

I wish that I am a giver but I lost everything, home, belongings, work energy and even the personal history. So, at least, I hope I can assist my students to overcome these horror, ordeals and calamities and to support my colleges to develop our professional career.

Contents

Foreword

Few Sudanese university Academics, especially in pharmacy, have become accustomed to engaging in scientific writing, especially working on issuing the methodological or reference books. Therefore, we have to express our salutes and gratitude to Dr. Abd ElRahman Mahmoud Gamil for issuing this useful book to all students of the Sudanese colleges of pharmacy.

This book, with its valuable content, is a useful scientific reference for pharmacy students who wish to future engagement in the field of industrial pharmacy. This book provides valuable scientific information about pharmaceutical packaging in general and about single-use injection manufacturing needs and techniques in specific. It clearly explains complete information about the importance of packaging as an approved basic prerequisite in registering pharmaceutical products and in explaining its importance to protect the product, its effectiveness is proven, the patient's shape and appearance are accepted, and its types. Also, the book briefed the important factors in choosing materials, ensuring quality, and contributing for adequate protection measures during shipping, transportation, storage and use by the patient.

As mentioned earlier, the importance of this book for students concerned and interested in working in pharmaceutical products' manufacturing. This is shown in the great experience of the author that he gained in his involvement as director of the first Sudanese factory specialized in the production of single-use syringes. The author experience was evident in the given precise manufacturing details of this strategic and important product, which is highly needed in many potential therapeutic interventions for many medical cases of extreme necessity.

To make the utmost use of this book, we recommend that the author carefully make an affordable availability of this book to the largest number of students in the colleges of pharmacy, and also encourage the continuous production of such useful scientific publications by other faculty colleagues.

Professor Mirghani Abd ElRahman Yousif
Former Dean of Faculty of Pharmacy
Former Dean of Scientific Affairs
Gezira University-Sudan
Taif University-KSA

Preface

A pharmaceutical product will not be registered to become a licensed pharmaceutical product and ready for distribution and patient-use unless it is presented in its final pack.

During the years in the pharmaceutical industry, I noticed a great care on the formulation, the production and the quality control activities, at the same time packaging was considered as a secondary task and not have the appropriate care. However, a proper and elegant packaging is the key factor for successful marketing and patient acceptability considering that without a proper packaging, all the efforts in production will go with the wind. There are many deficiencies is QA and QC for the packaging material at the level of the finished products factories. Also, I noticed a lack of knowledge in the pharmaceutical sector; professional and student, regarding the technology of dispausable syringes which is a very critical element in the field of patient care and health providing.

My students always asking me for a comprehensive, concise and simple reference for the subject.

During these years of war at my country, I tried to gather the information I have gained during my professional life and university teaching and support them with the relative diagrams and figures to ease the studying of the subject.

The book is divided into five sections:

1. General packaging container-closure systems.

2. The QA of packaging container-closure systems.

3. The quality control tests.

4. Technology of single-use plastic syringes.

5. the requirements and tests for single-use plastic syringes.

I hope this book may hit the goals and may be helpful and of value for the targeted groups.

Dr. A. M. Gamil

Section 1:

Introduction to Packaging Materials and Container–Closure Systems

1.1 Introduction

A pharmaceutical formulation is considered to be bulk until it packed in a suitable container, labelled and contained in a suitable box then it becomes a pharmaceutical product as shown in (figure1-1).

Figure 1-1 Examples of packed pharmaceutical products

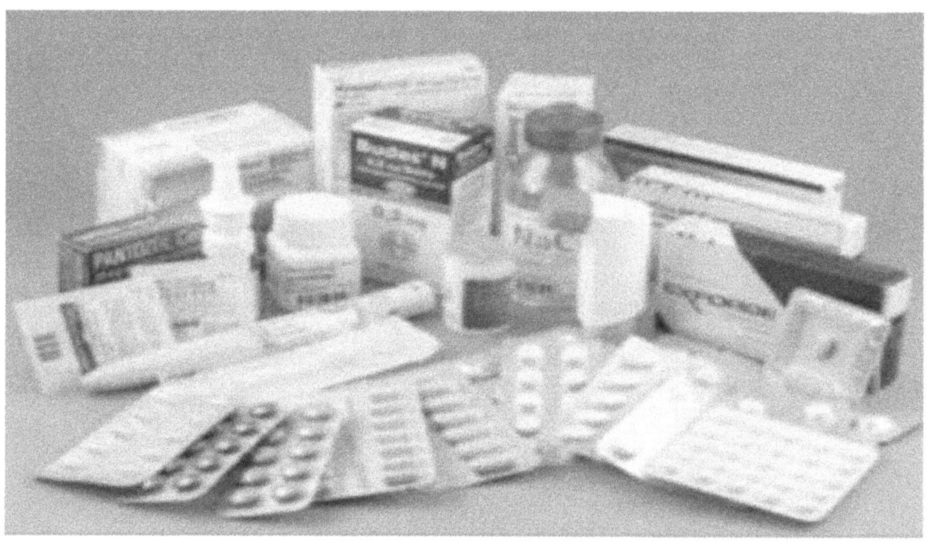

The pack provides the following functions

Packaging is the process of appropriately placing a pharmaceutical preparation in a suitable container to retain it effect and potency until be consumed.

Packaging can be defined as an art and science of presenting a pharmaceutical dosage form in such a way that it will be appropriately stored, handled, transported and easy to use. It helps in protection, identification and elegant presentation of the product to provide convenience and user acceptability and allows a place to provide the required information and instructions. This requires the use of the following apartments:

1- Container.

2- Closure system.

3- Carton or outer pack.

4- Box, cardboard. and may need other outer packs.

1.2 Functions of Packaging

1- Containment of the product.

2- Identification of the product.

3- Information which is written on the pack.

4- Allow appropriate storage status.

5- Protection of the product during handling and shipment.

6- Elegant presentation.

7- Convenience.

8- Allow safe distribution.

9- Ease of administration.

10- Efficacy, safety and uniformity of the product.

11- Reproducibility, integrity, purity and stability.

12- Branding and anti-counterfeiting, giving the product its specific presentation.

1.3 Requirements for a Suitable Packaging Material and Container

1- The container should have appropriate protection of the product from the surrounding hazards which include:

   ☞   Light mostly for those light sensitive products.

   ☞   Temperature to an acceptable extend.

   ☞   Moisture; which greatly affects the stability.

   ☞   Gases like oxygen and carbon dioxide.

   ☞   Protect the product from viable and non-viable contamination.

2- It should provide sufficient mechanical strength to withstand the vibration which is usually takes during transportation. It is required to resist compression during storage, compaction and dropping.

3- It should be capable to minimize abrasion that may produce electrostatic charges which may affect the stability.

4- It should prevent product loss or gain any foreign material and should prevent ingress and shed of particles.

5- Minimum allowed leaching.

6- It shall be elegant and presentable appearance to satisfy the market and patient needs.

7- It should be easily to label and can provide quick identification of the product.

8- It should be cheap and of economic feasibility.

9- It should be convenient and use to use the patient.

10- Must be non-toxic and non-reactive with the content and should not provide any taste or odor to the product.

11- Have a good adaptability to the modern high-speed production lines.

12- Must meet applicable tamper-resistance requirement and Drug Regulatory Authority approved.

1.4 Types of Pharmaceutical Packaging

❋ **Primary pack:**

This is the packaging which in direct contact with the product or the dosage form (tablet, capsule, liquid, semisolid or injection…. etc)

❋ **Secondary pack:**

Carton box to contain the primary pack, ancillary components, cups, spoons, leaflet …*etc.*

❋ Hard carton boxes to contain the individual group of packs.

1.4.1 Primary Pack

Powders, granules, tablets, capsules, semisolids as creams, ointments, gels, lotions, shampoos, liquids as solutions, suspensions and powder for reconstitution, emulsions, some of which are sterile.

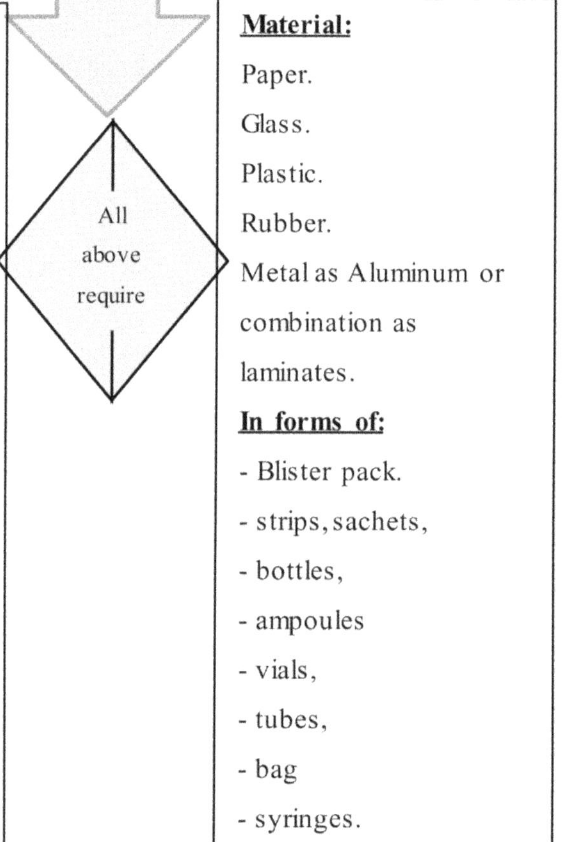

Design of the primary pack:

. Child resistant, easy to use by the elder.

. Tamper proof to guard against pilferages and contamination.

. Compatible with the content, minimum sorption and leaching.

. Enable product stability.

. protect the product against the atmospheric oxygen, light, moisture, CO_2, temperature, pests, rodents, particulate and microorganism.

Material:

Paper.

Glass.

Plastic.

Rubber.

Metal as Aluminum or combination as laminates.

In forms of:

- Blister pack.

- strips, sachets,

- bottles,

- ampoules

- vials,

- tubes,

- bag

- syringes.

- Multiple doses or single dose.

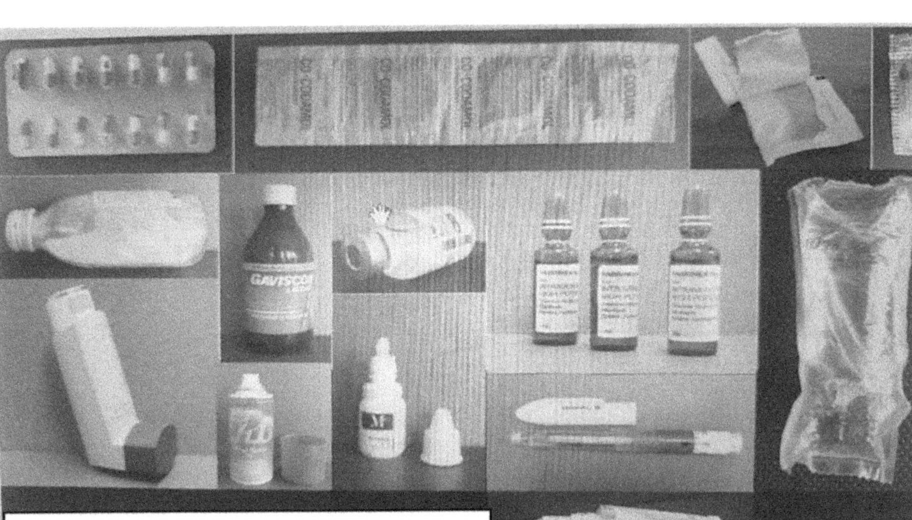

Figure 1-2 Different primary packaging forms

1.4.2 Secondary Pack

The secondary packaging has many functions as mentioned before. It gives protection for the product in the primary pack against atmospheric factors. It is the packaging of the primary packaging containing the product.

It provides additional protection against mechanical hazards, shock, dropping, vibration and abrasion during handling and transport. It gives the product the elegant and respectful presentation. Secondary pack aid in differentiation between the various brands and assist in identification of product during dispensing and use by the patient.

Figure 1-3 Examples of secondary packaging

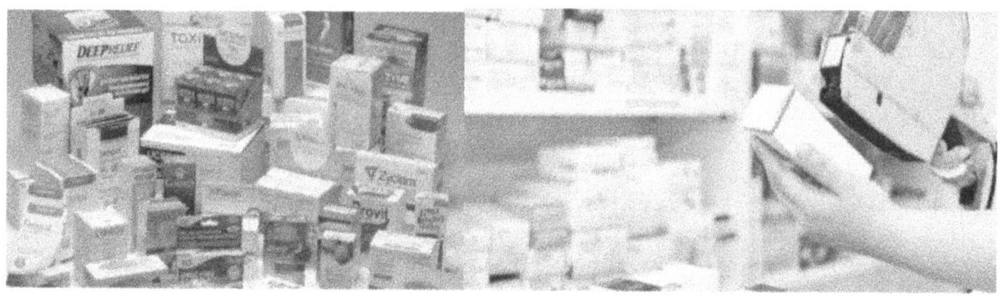

Table 1-1 Examples of primary and secondary

Type	Material	Examples
Primary Packaging	Glass	Bottles, ampoules, vials
	Plastic	Ampoules, vials, IV bags, bottles, dropper bottles
Secondary packaging	Plastic	Wrappers
	Cardboard	Boxes
	Paper	Labels, PP papers strips, leaflet

1.5 Containers

Primary containers are in direct contact with the preparation

And the also the closure. Thus, quality of the container is of great importance and should fulfil the following requirements:

☞ It should be neutral, non-toxic and non-reactive with the formulation it contains.

☞ It should protect the preparation from any environmental hazards to maintain the stability of the content. It should be made of material that can withstand the handling processes, pressure and temperature.

1.5.1 Types of Containers

Containers can be divided according to the closure system, according to the administration method and according to the material and material properties:

1. Well-closed containers:

    Containers that prevent leakage of content during transportation and handling.

2. Device pack containers:

    These are devices used to administer it content directly in the route of administration as the prefilled syringe and transdermal delivery system.

3. Light-resistant containers:

    These containers block the light to reach the content. It is used for light sensitive products.

4. Multi-dose containers:

    These are containers that hold the content to be delivered in various doses at different interval without changes in the strength, purity and quality of the remaining portion. Multi-dose containers are used for injectable preparation being contain in vials.

5. Single-dose containers:

These are containers containing only one single dose as in parenteral preparations. However, unit-dose containers mag give the function but includes oral administration which are suitable for instable product and avoiding medication errors in providing the accurate dose and convenience of the patient.

6. Air-tight containers:

Hermetic containers are sealed so as to prevent ingress of air, particulate and moisture providing complete protection for the product.

7. Aerosol containers:

These containers should have sufficient mechanical strength so as to withstand the internal pressure of the aerosol.

1.6 Closures

Closures is a part of the container that it provides a good complete seal for the container and should be compatible with the product and suitable and acceptable for the patient use.

It should provide a suitable seal for ingress of microbes.

Closures are available in five basic designs:

1- Screw-on, threaded or lug.

2- Crimp-on (crowns).

3- Press-on (snap).

4- Roll-on.

5- Friction.

1.6.1 Screw-On, Threaded or Lug

The threads of the cap fill the thread gaps in the neck of the bottle (male/female) style figure (1-4). The liner in the cap is pressed by the top surface of the bottle neck providing a seal to the bottle opening and thus protects the product and prevent leakage of content (figure 1-5). Screw cap is generally made of Aluminum metal plate or tin plates or thermosetting and thermoplastic types of plastic.

Figure (1-4): Threads of the bottle neck

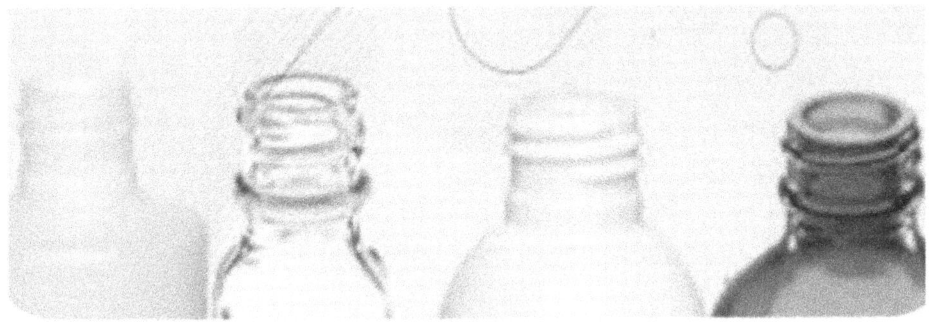

Figure 1-5: Threads of the cap and liner

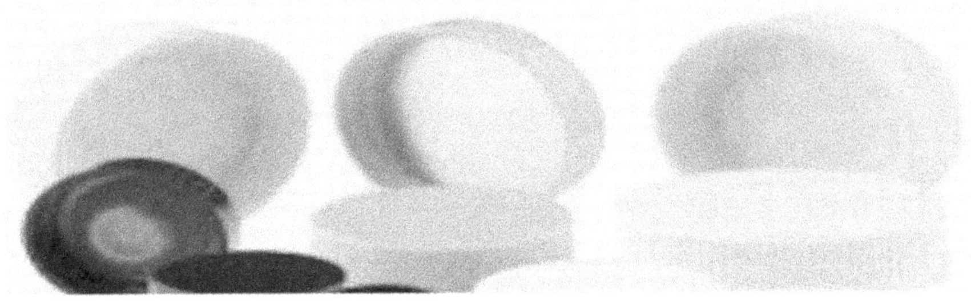

Lug is the same but the threads are not continuous, gaps are there interrupting the threads. It requires on quarter circle turn.

1.6.2 Crimp on (Crown)

Used for the closure of beverage, generally made of metal figure 1-6.

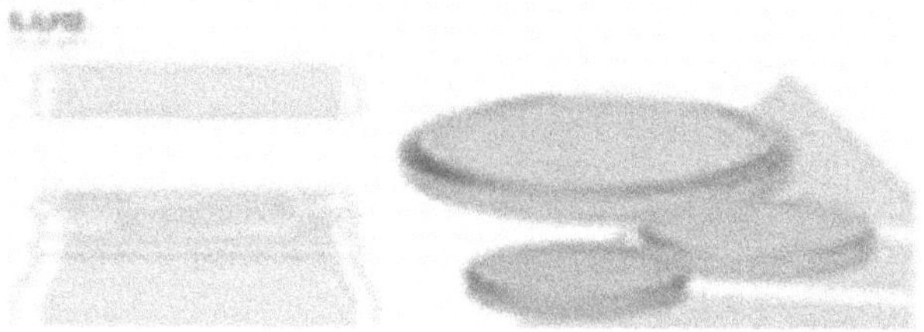

1.6.3 Roll-On Closures

The aluminum roll or lacquered tinplate cap for sealing of a narrow neck. The unthread cap is moulded on to the neck of a bottle and forms an air-tight seal. Cap can be seal securely, opened easily and resealed effectively figure 1-7.

Resealable and non-resealable closures are available for use in glass or plastic bottles.

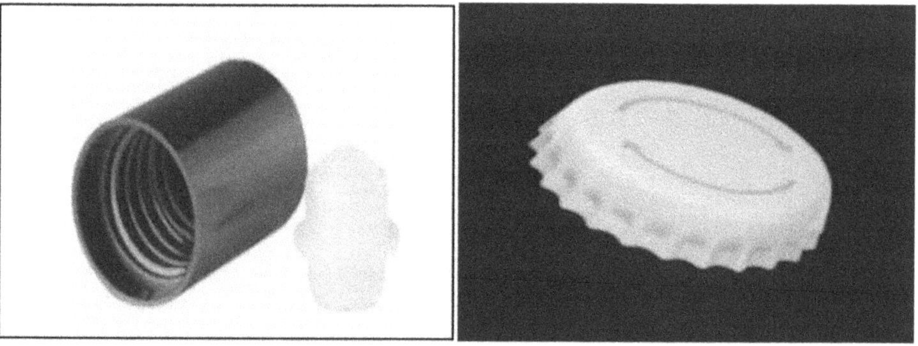

Figure 1-7 Roll-on closure   Figure 1-6 crimp on (crown)

1.6.4 Pilfer Proof Closure

This closure a longer length than roll-on closure. The additional length goes under the lower last thread of the bottle and keeping attached to the upper part. On opening the bottle, it detached from the upper part of the cap and remains as a ring around the neck of the bottle under the last thread, figure 1-8.

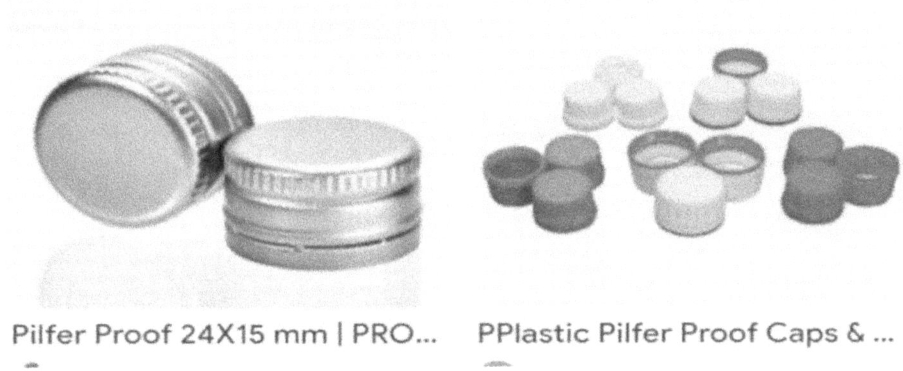

Figure 1-8 Pilfer Proof caps

1.6.5 Closure Liners

Closure liner can be defined as that material being inserted in the cap to seal between the cap and the container opening. It is made of resilient backing and a facing material. The backing material must be soft enough to take up any irregularities in the surface and elastic enough to recover the original shape when removed and replaced. It may be homogeneous of one plastic material or heterogeneous of different backing and facing materials.

Required properties of liner:

➤ Should be inert and compatible with the product.

> ➤ Should be re-closable and effectively sealed and of enough thickness.

> ➤ Should have a low gas/ vapor transmission rate.

> ➤ Should provide an optimum torque to remove the cap.

> ➤ Should be heat-resistant and thermostable to withstand autoclaving.

> ➤ Should not be changed during storage.

> ➤ Should be compatibles with the high-speed production operations.

> ➤ Elegant and harmonious with the container.

> ➤ Should be cheap.

Materials of liners:

Rubber, Plastic, Glass, Metal, Cork.

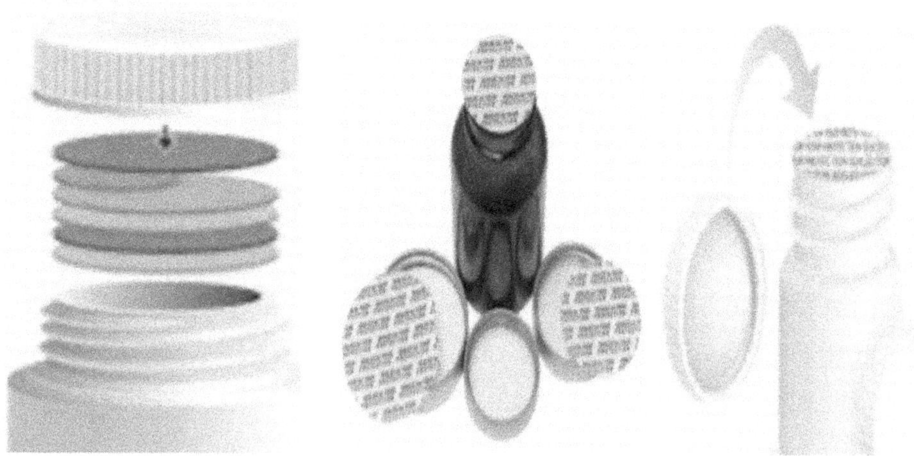

Figure 1-9 Closure liners Overlock liner.

1.6.6 Stopper, Lid, Top or Cap.

Stopper shall have the following properties:

- Must be inert, compatible with content and protectant.

- Should be sterile for parenteral vials.

- Must provide good seal with the container to prevent leakage.

- Snug fit between the inner surface of the closure and outer face of the container.

- Easy to open and easy to close.

- Allow good grip when opening by twisting.

  - ✓ Metal is used in parenteral vials and plastic is used in the form of Thermosets and Thermoplastics.

  - ✓ Tubes are closed at one end by metal and the other by folding.

1.7 Packaging Material

Glass and plastics are the most commonly used packaging material. Although laminates and papers are used as primary packaging materials. Papers and cartons a commonly used as secondary packaging. Table 1-2 shows the commonly used materials.

Table 1-2 Description of common packaging materials

Material	Description
Glass	☞ Type I: borosilicate glass ☞ Type II: treated soda lime glass. ☞ Type III: regular soda lime glass. ☞ Type NP: general purpose soda lime glass. ☞ Colored glass
Metal	Tin, Iron, Aluminum, Lead.
Plastics	☞ Thermosetting resins: phenolic, urea, ☞ Thermoplastic resins: polyethylene, polypropylene, PVC, polystyrene, polycarbamide, polyamide (Nylon), polyethylene terephthalate.
Rubber	☞ Normal rubber. ☞ Neoprene rubber. ☞ Butyl rubber.
laminates	Multiple polyethylene layers joined together by way of lamination barrier layer made of aluminum or EVOH (ethylene vinyl alcohol) polymer.
Paper	PP film coated paper and hard cardboard.

1.7.1 Factor Determining the Selection of Material

- ✓ The dosage form and route of administration and status of the targeted patient.

- ✓ Product stability and excipients characteristics.

- ✓ Terminal sterilization to withstand the elevated temperature.

- ✓ Allow visual inspection.

- ✓ Compatibility with content.

- ✓ Convenience, aesthetics, presentation to the market and the authority, cost and environment friendship.

- ✓ For parenteral product it should maintain sterility and prevent contamination.

- ✓ Ease of pourability and withdrawal of semisolid preparations.

- ✓ Sensitivity of the product to light.

- ✓ Patient acceptability.

- ✓ Channels of distribution, where, when, how, by whom is to be used or administered?

- ✓ Transportation vehicles and route of distribution.

- ✓ The available facilities at the site of production.

1.7.2 Glass

Generally, glass is the more preferable packaging material.

What is glass?

☞ Glass is composed from silicon dioxide (Sand), Sodium Carbonate (Soda ash), Calcium Carbonate (lime stone), Cullet (broken glass), Aluminum, Boron, Potassium, Magnesium, Zinc and Barium.

Advantages of glass:

1- Glass is hygienic and can withstand sterilization heat.

2- It is inert, non-reactive depending on its type.

3- Can adapt high speed lines.

4- Suitable for various closures

5- Favorable protection for the contents.

6- Can be transparent or dark coloured.

7- Glass is easily to be labeled.

Disadvantages of glass:

1- Fragile and easy to break.

2- Release alkali to aqueous preparations.

3- Heavy to carry.

Synthesis of glass:

1- Sand (silica) heated with limestone (Calcium Carbonate) and soda ash (Sodium Carbonate) heated to 1500 °C in a furnace.

2- Ingredients melt and form a homogeneous mass.

This mass converted to glass by;

a- Blow moulding; blowing molten glass using compressed air and moulding into a cavity of a metal mold.

b- In drawing: molten glass is pulled through the die or rollers that shape the soft glass.

c- Pressing: mechanical force presses the molten glass against the walls of the mold.

d- Casting by using centrifugal force to distributed the molten glass to sides of the mold.

Tubular glass fabrication:

Molten glass converted into glass tubing and then the tubing is cut to produce individual tubes which are then converted to ampoules or vials.

Additives to glass to improve its properties:

☞ Alumina (Al_2O_3) to increase hardness.

☞ Selenium or Cobalt oxide to improve clarity.

☞ Lead Oxide gives clarity and sparkle but make the glass soft.

☞ Boron: increase the thermal resistant.

☞ Arsenic oxide to prevent blistering.

☞ Amber to protect from light.

☞ Green for beverage.

☞ Opaque white gives prestige to toiletries and cosmetics.

☞ Colours are added as in Table 1-3.

Is glass inert?

glass is inert but not totally so.

It contains;

Silica 59 – 71%

Calcium oxide 5 – 12%.

Sodium oxide 12 – 17%.

Alumina 0.5 – 3%

Traces of ferric oxide, titanium dioxide, potassium and Magnesium oxides. So, leaching may occur, sodium increases the alkalinity content.

Under fluctuated temperature and humidity, salts of glass accumulate on the surface "blooming" which is undesirable.

To reduce the leaching, glass can be soaked in hot water or dilute acid.

Glass surface can be treated by Sulphur to make it resistant to water or acidic medium.

Table 1-3 Materials of added colours

Colour	Material
Amber	Iron oxides, manganese, carbon oxides and sulphar compounds
Brown	Iron oxides, carbon oxides and sulphar compounds and Manganese dioxide.
Green	Iron oxides, manganese dioxide, chromium dioxide.
Yellow green	Uranium oxides
Deep blue	Cobalt oxides, Copper dioxides.
Light blue	Copper compounds
Yellow	Lead with antimony, Cadmium and Sulphar.
Reds	Gold chloride, selenium and copper compounds.
Amethyst	Manganese oxides
Black	Mix manganese, cobalt and iron.
White	Tin compounds, antimony oxides.

1.7.2.1 Types of glass

Glass type I

Glass type II

Glass type III

Glass type NP

<u>Glass types I</u>

Neutral glass, borosilicate glass (Silicon Dioxide and Boron). Produced by adding boron oxide to glass; borosilicate glass.

<u>Advantages of type I glass:</u>

The best pharmaceutical grade of high hydrolytic resistance.

Most inert, least amount of leaching.

Lowest coefficient thermal expansion.

<u>Disadvantages:</u>

Most expensive because it has a high glass transition temperature, so needed complicated process.

<u>Uses of type I glass:</u>

- Suitable for packing of all pharmaceutical products; solid dosage forms, semisolid dosage form, liquid dosage form, LVP & SVP ampoule and vials.

- It contains the least or no leachable alkali oxides.

Glass type II

Standard material, soda lime glass + sodium carbonate to decrease the glass transition temperature, but this increased water solubility, and Calcium Oxide is added to increase the hydraulic resistance. The surface is treated by sulphar dioxide, washout sodium sulphate. Treated soda lime glass is suitable for solution of pH less than 7. At pH more than 7, leaches oxides.

This is the second-grade glass.

Advantages:

→ Lower melting point than type I.

→ Cheaper and easier production process.

→ Because of the treated surface, it possesses an appropriate hydraulic resistance.

Disadvantages:

→ Cannot be used for parenteral preparations of pH less than 7 because it contains basic oxides which will increase the pH and consequently affects the stability of the content.

Uses:

→ Type II glass is used for packing the aqueous preparation.

→ Can be used for ophthalmic solutions and other dropper bottles and other pharmaceutical preparations,

Type III (Regular Soda lime Glass)

→ This type is composed of commercial sodalime and is not treated but it has a better resistance than the commercial type.

→ It renders the aqueous content alkaline due to it high content of alkali oxides.

→ It flakes and separate easily.

Uses:

→ Used for packing solid dosage forms.

→ For non-aqueous preparations.

→ Used in food packaging.

→ For large volumes.

Type NP (General Purpose Soda Lime Glass)

→ This type is made of soda lime general grade and is none parenteral glass. It is the lowest grade of glass.

Uses:

→ Suitable for large volume of topical products as mouth washes.

1.7.3 Plastics

The British Standard Institute defines plastic as a wide range of solid composite material mostly organic material, usually based on synthetic resins or modified polymers of natural origin and possessing appreciable mechanical strength. At a certain stage of processing most plastics can be casted, molded or polymerized directly into a shape.

There are many uses for plastic in packaging of different dosage forms. For example, bottles are used for solids and liquid products, tubes for creams, ointments and gels. The pouches are used for the individual suppositories. Blister packs are used for packaging of tablets and capsule. I.V bags, bottles and containers for TPN. Jars are used for lotions and shampoos. Overwraps are used to wrap up packs and containers.

Commonly used plastic for packaging:

Polyethylene. PE, Polypropylene PP, Polyethylene terephthalate, Polyamides (Nylon), polystyrene, Polyvinylchloride PVC. Polyvinylidene chloride, Polycarbonates.

1.7.3.1 Properties of plastic

- Light, shatterproof.

- Can be clear or opaque.

- Easily shaped, sealed and designed.

- Allow inclusion of acids.

- Squeezable.

- Less resistant to heat.

- Leachable components.

- Permeability problems.

- Long time exposure to oxygen and light make it brittle and easy to break.

1.7.3.2 Plastic Synthesis

Polymers are produced by addition reaction or condensation reaction of monomers.

The product is:

Copolymer: more than one type of monomer or,

Homopolymer: contains one type of monomer.

Types of polymers:

A. Thermosetting plastic: cross-linked structure.

B. Thermoplastic polymer: linear and branched polymer chain.

1.7.3.3 Thermosetting Plastic

Thermoset polymer can only be shaped once due to its cross-linking structure which cannot flow.

Urea aldehyde, epoxides, Urethanes, unsaturated polyesters and melamine.

Advantage of plastic:

- Cheaper than glass.

- Easy to transport and light in weight.

- No risk of breakage.

- Flexible.

Disadvantage:

- Chemically not inert as type I glass.

- Having some permeability to gases and water vapor.

- Possessing electrostatic charge that may lead to accumulation of particles.

Uses:

- Rigid bottles for tablets and capsules.

- Squeezable bottles for drops and nasal sprays.

- Flexible tubes, jars, strips and blisters.

1.7.3.4 Thermoplastics

Melt at high temperature and become liquid then can be molded into various shapes as bottles, tubes, film …. etc.

Then can be softened, melted again and molded many times.

PET, Polystyrene, PP, Nylon, Polyester, PVC and Polycarbonates.

Employed in BFS in the manufacture of IV fluids as shown in diagram 1-10.

Figure 1-10: diagrammatic presentation of BFS process

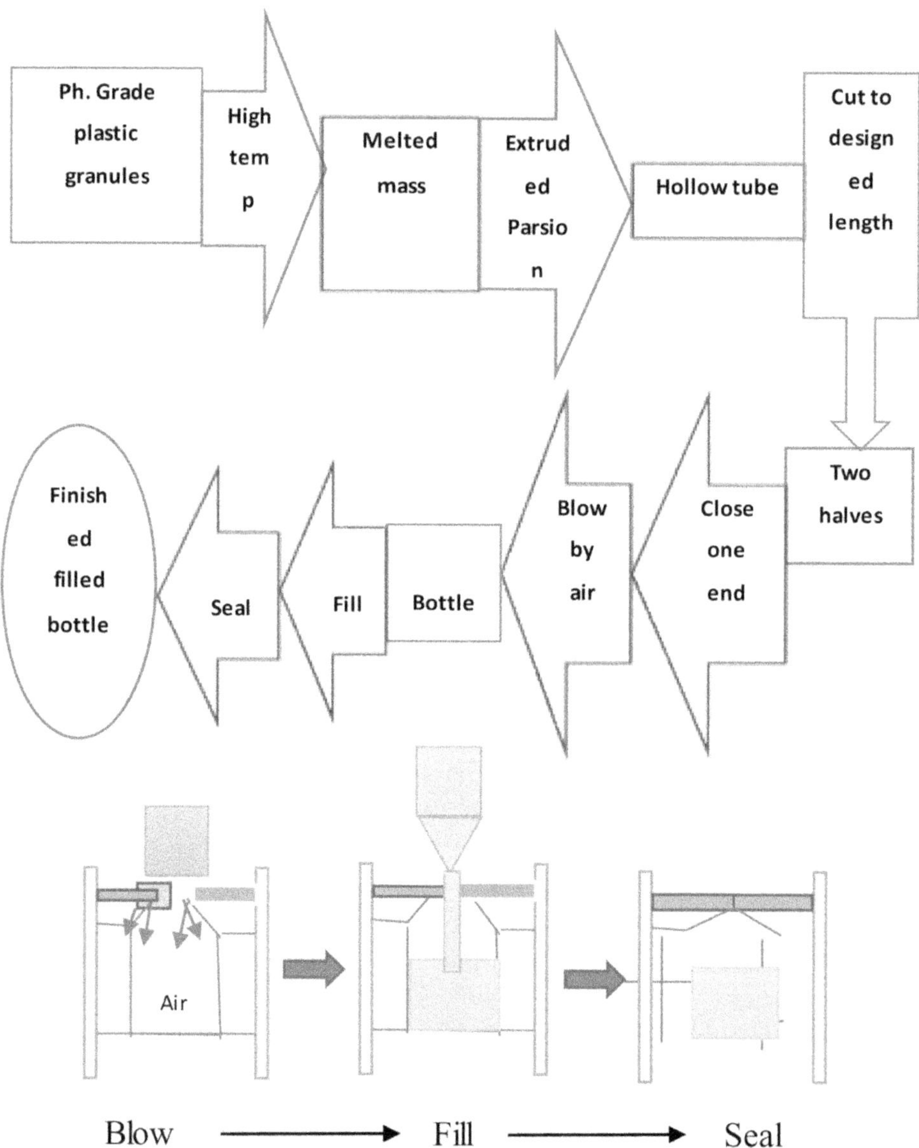

Figure 1-11 products of BFS

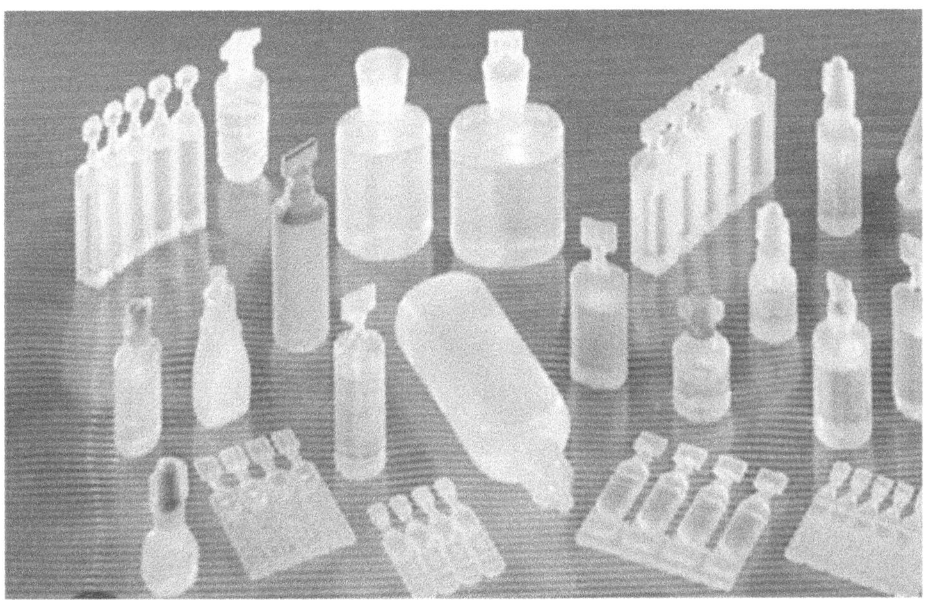

1-Polyethylene PE:

There are two types of polyethylene, high density polyethylene HDPE and low density poly ethylene LDPE. PE is widely used in pharmaceutical packaging because of its toughness and resistance to moisture. Chemically inert, low cost, easily processing and its electrical insulation properties. It is flexible and easily to be sealed.

Limitations:

x   Lack of rigidity and low softening point.

x   Low tensile strength.

x   Prone to oxidation.

x   Cracking due to stress in the presence of surfactant or oils.

    x   Considerable permeability to gases and water moisture according to the density. HDPE is less permeable than LDPE.

2-Polypropylene:

It is semi-rigid. Translucent tough and has good chemical resistance and cracking when pressed. It possesses a good heat resistance property making it suitable for sterilization. It is colorless, odorless with excellent tensile strength even at high temperature. It is resistant to alkies and acids. It has a low permeability to water vapour, but its permeability to gases is between HDPE and PVC being used for containers and I.V bottles.

3-Polystyrene:

Polystyrene is versatile, clear and non-toxic. Light in weight and good dimensional stability. It is easily foamed (styrene foam). It is used for jars for ointments and creams of low water content.

Limitations:

Some chemicals like isopropyl myristate produce crazing which is a fine cracks network on the surface followed by weakening and collapse of the container.

4-Polyvinyl chloride PVC:

It is versatile, considerable strength/toughness, easy to blend and have good resistance to grease and oils. It is resistant to chemicals and having good clarity.

It is used as a hard packaging material in the main components of the IV fluids sets.

Limitation:

Poor press and compression resistance which may be improved by addition of elastomer but it increases the permeability.

5-Polyvinylidene chloride:

PVDC is an excellent moisture barrier, water vapor, UV light, odors, inorganic alkalis and acids. Resistant to chemical aqueous solutions, aliphatic hydrocarbons, fatty acids and detergents. It possesses a good thermoform capabilities. PVDC is cost effective in coating and can be customized according to the barrier requirement. The medical grade is non-toxic and of high level of transparency which provides an aesthetical presentation to the product.

1.7.3.5 Problems related to plastic packaging:

A packaging system should protect the content without altering the quality of the product until the last dose is removed.

The problems associated with the plastic packaging are:

1- Leaching.

2- Permeation.

3- Sorption.

4- Chemical reaction.

5- Alternation.

Leaching:

Additives to some plastic to improve some properties may find a way to leach out into the container content. Couring materials of plastic may add traces of colour to the drug product contained in plastic containers. Leaching of dyes to parenteral preparations may be harmful.

Permeability:

Permeation is the transmission of gases, water vapor or liquids through the walls of the product container. The major problem is the permeation of water vapour and oxygen into the product container which may lead to hydrolysis and oxidation respectively. Volatile ingredients may exchange into or out of the product.

Figure 1-12 Water Vapor Permeation of various Packaging Materials

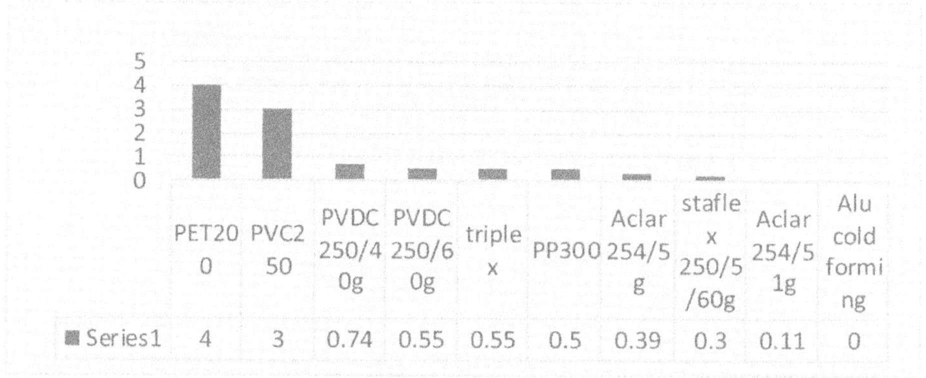

Sorption

Sorption is the phenomenon of removal of the drug constituents in packaging container by the surface of walls of the container. This may result in altering the physical and chemical characteristics of the products. Leading to decrease in the therapeutic action, changing the structure of the ingredients to non-active substances or induction of degradation.

Change in pH and other physiochemical changes may be associated.

Chemical reactivity

Plastic ingredients or additives that being added to stabilize the plastic material may react with one or more of the components of the content, additive and their function are illustrated in table 1-4. This incompatibility may result in physical or chemical changes to either the drug constituents or to the plastic of the container resulting in untoward outcomes.

Alternation

This is a physical or chemical change modifying the plastic structure and mechanical properties caused by the contents. Oils softens the PE and hydrocarbons attack PE and PVC.

Table 1-4 Plastic Additives & Processing Aids

Material	Function
Phthalate ester	Plasticizer
Talc	Filler, extender.
Rubber to polystyrene	Toughening agent
Calcium-zinc salts to PVC	Stabilizer
Cresol	Antioxidant
Substituted phenol	UV absorber
Titanium dioxide	Opacifier
Ultramarine pigment and dyes	Whitener
Pigments and dyes	Colouring materials
Wax, liquid paraffin	Lubricating agents
Metal stearates, silicon oil	Lubrication for the mould.
Amides, finely divided silica	Slip agents to avoid sticking together.
Surfactant	To reduce static accumulation of plastic.

1.7.3.6 Comparison between the commonly used plastic types in Pharmaceutical industry

Property	PE(HDPE&LDPE)	PP	PVC
General	Compatible, HDP is widely used	Contain less additives	Many additives
Sorption	Can sorb material	Less sorption	Replaced by other types
Appearance	Milky, translucent, strong and stiff	Clear	Clear, glossy and flexible
Heat	HDPE can be autoclaved	Resistant to heat, withstand sterilization	Heat sensitive
Moisture	HDPE good barrier, LDPE is poor	Excellent barrier	Fair
Gases	Permeable	Better odor barrier	Poor to medium
Oils	Permeable	More resistant to grease and oils	Excellent barrier
Cost	cheep	cheep	Cheep

1.7.4 Rubber and Elastomers

Rubber is used as stopper closure on parenteral containers. It allows hypodermic needle to enter the container and reseal when the needle is removed. It is soft enough to mould and conform the container opening allowing tight seal. Rubbers are formulation of elastomers that contains 2-10 additives. Elastomers are naturally extracted from rubber tree or from petrochemicals.

1.7.4.1 Composition of rubber

Butyl, chlorobutyl, silicon,chloroprene and nitrile elastomers are synthetic rubber. Natural rubber is mixed with chlorobutyl to help resist corning in closure and let it withstand multiple penetration of needle. Rubber has some permeability, leaching and sorption properties.

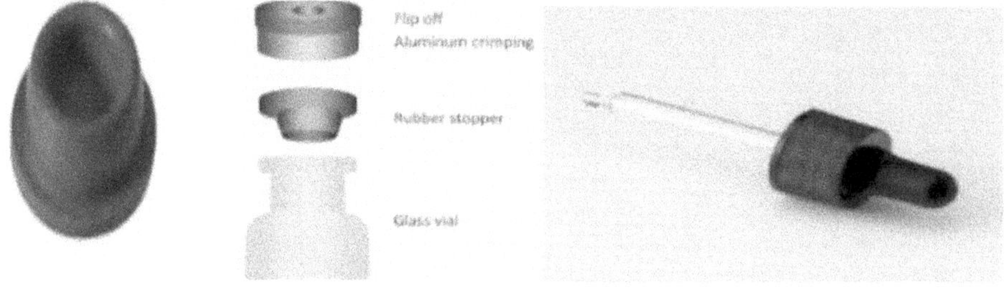

1.7.4.2 Synthesis of rubber

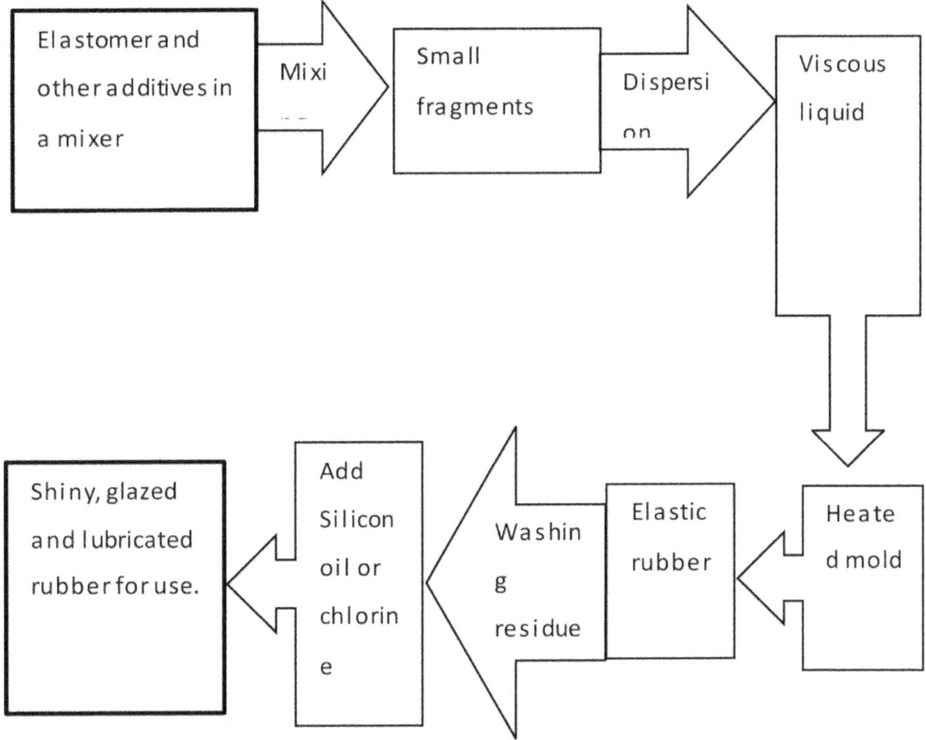

Figure 1-13 synthesis of rubber

1.7.5 Metal

Metal is widely used for packaging pharmaceutical products other than parenteral preparation. It is strong, impermeable to gases, moisture, water vapor, volatile aroma, light and microorganisms. It is a shutter proof and strong to withstand pressurized preparations. It is resistant to various temperature levels. Metal is used as tubes, blisters, sheets and foils, cans, gas cylinders, aerosols and for tamper proof containers. Aluminum, tin, lead and iron are the commonly used metals. Tinplate sheet is steal coated with a thin deposit of tin. Used for cans, MDI containers, tubes for cream, ointment, gel, pouches for granules, liquid suppositories, blister bags and closures. It is mechanically strong, shatterproof, light weight, impermeable, malleable. Malleability allow the metal collar to be crimped in place.

To isolate metal from the content, it will be coated with vinyl, acrylic or epoxy. The outer metal is coated to enable printing.

When squeezed it will not return to its place, so it will not suck oxygen. Metals can be coated to allow printing.

Figure 1-14 Aluminum foil for packaging

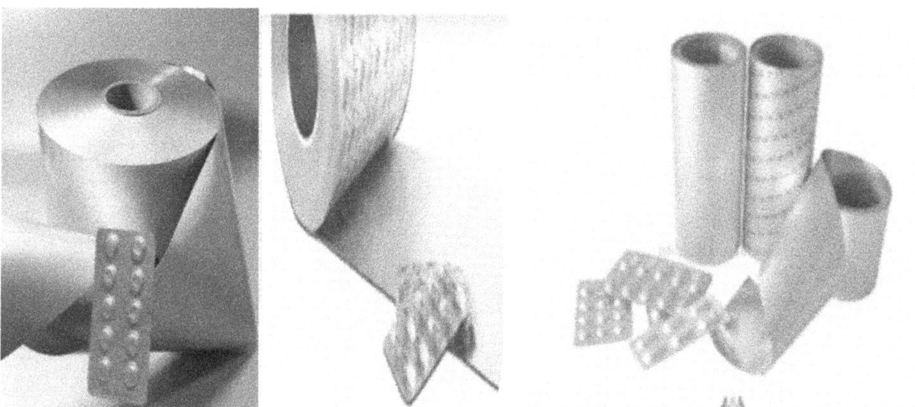

1.7.5.1 Aluminum

- Light in comparison with other metals.

- Barrier to light, gases and chemicals.

- Impermeable to gases, water vapor and moisture.

- Hard containers as collapsible tubes for semisolids, cans, aerosol containers, tubes for effervescent tablets.

- Aluminum foil or sheet is widely used in blisters for tablets and capsule.

- Aluminum can be formed in a variety of forms and shapes depending on its thickness.

- Aluminum can be coated with epoxide, vinyl and phenolic to guard against corrosion at extreme pH.

1.7.5.2 Tin

As it is expensive it is generally used to coat lead and other metals because it is resistant to chemical reactions. Tin-coated lead tubes combines the softness of lead and the inertness of tin. It is used for packing of food materials and ophthalmic ointment tubes.

1.7.5.3 Lead

Lead is cheaper than the other metals, it possesses a considerable toxicity known as lead poisoning. It is soft, the tubes are fragile depending on the thickness. It is used in tooth paste tubes after internal coating with epoxy or inert polymer.

1.7.5.4 Iron

For pharmaceutical use it should be coated by tin due to its rapid corrosion.

1.7.6 Papers

Labels, leaflets, cartons, bags, sacks and sachets.

It is not generally used as primary pack except when coated.

Low cost, non-toxic, easily recycled, easy to torn or cut or open.

Ability to hold grease, leaflet in patient information, strength and rigid cartons, easy to print and coat.

Tailor-made opacity, colour, porosity.

No barrier properties, moisture, gas and odour. It is moisture sensitive.

No heat or cold seal unless it is coated.

Low transparency.

* Paper can be coated by polymer or laminated to plastic or Aluminum foil. Polypaper OLB (opaque lamination base) is used for tablet strips figure 1-15.

Figure 1-15 Tablet paper strips

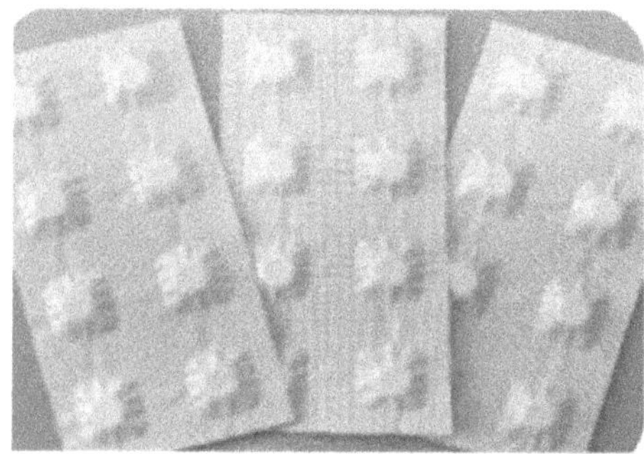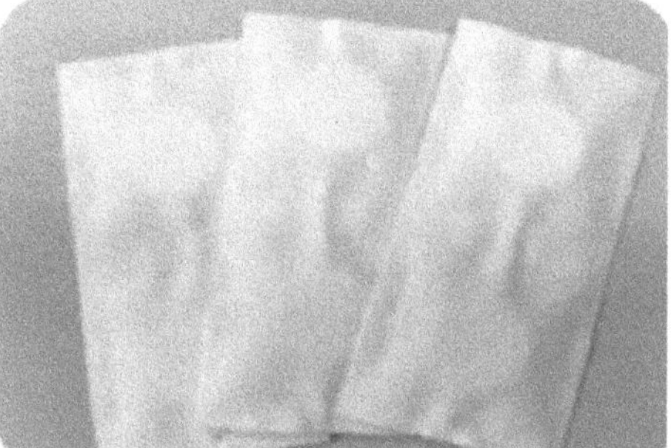

1.7.7 Fibrous Material

This includes papers and leaflets, labels, boxes, cartons, outer bags, trays, corners and base of pallets. It provides a good protection for the product and a safe stacking and an orgized stock display. Boxes include the drug, leaflets and spoons or measuring devices. Solid or corrugated board being wrapped by cellophane ease the shipment. Trays provide a good protection for bottles.

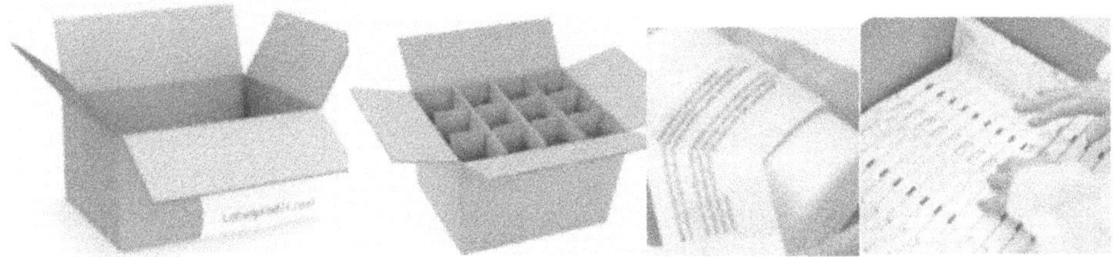

Figure 1-16 fibrous packaging material

1.7.8 Wrapping Material

These are materials used to wrap the box, the carton and even the pallet covering and protect it from dirt and water and to present an acceptable delivery. It may be thin transparent sheet or thick bubble wrap made of cellophane, rayophane or even paper.

Figure 1-17 wrapping sheets

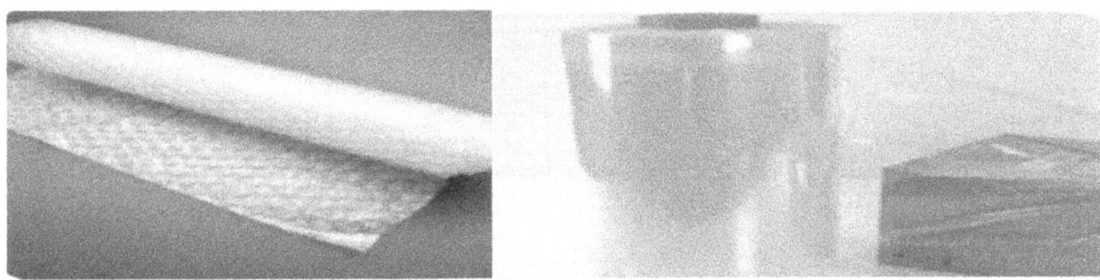

1.7.9 Laminates

Laminates are bonding of several interconnected layers of different materials. Each individual layer has its own specifications. The more the layers the more expensive is the product. It is protective to the content from gases, light and vapor.

Aluminum Barrier Laminate ALB, a thin layer of Aluminum layer is enclosed between two plastic layers providing a better protection. Polyethylene Barrier Laminate has multiple layers of HDPE including a barrier of ethylene vinyl alcohol to provide protection to the content and prolong the container life. Ethylene vinyl alcohol is a copolymer of optimum barrier characteristics.

Laminates are used to produce pharmaceutical packs as sachets, blisters, tubes, pouches…figure 1-17 etc.

Role of layers of laminate

Layer	Paper	Metal foil	PE
Functions	Strength	Barrier to moisture, gas, and light	Flexibility, heat sealability
	Easy to tear		
	Printability		

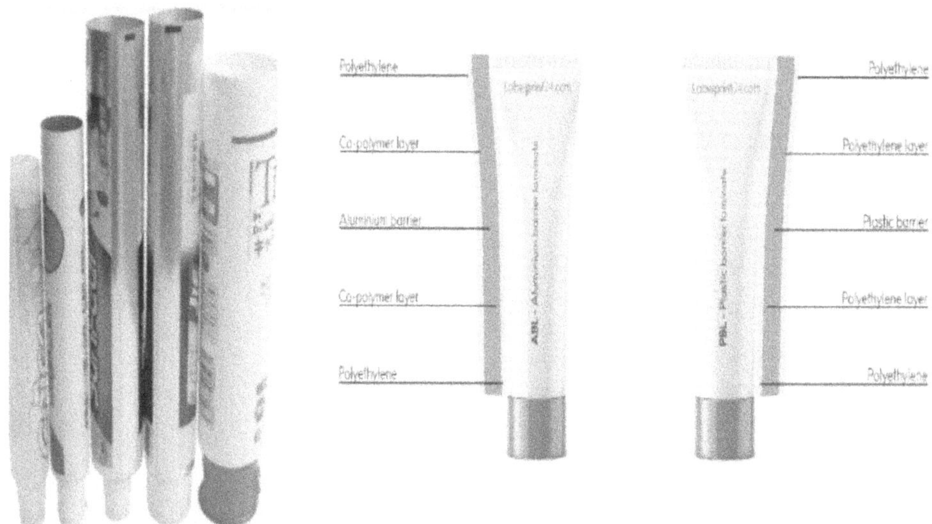

Figure 1-18 laminate tube *[Primepac, labelprint24.com]*

1.7.10 Tamper Proof Packaging

A tamper resistant packaging is the application of an evident indicator or barrier which should be removed or ruptured in order to access the content. So, if this indicator is ruptured or removed that means this is an evident that this container had been tampered. It is a security seal.

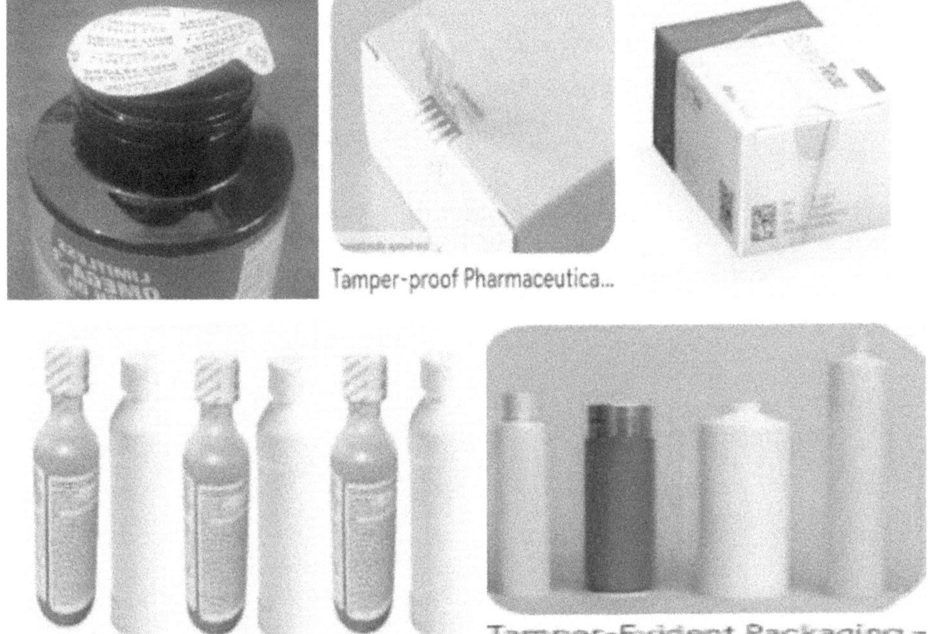

The following example in table 1-15 are considered to be tamper-proof.

Table 1-5 The followings are considered to be tamper-proof:

Item	Uses	Description
Blister pack	Tablets and capsules	
Strip packaging	Tablets and capsules	
Bubble pack	Tablets, capsule and others	
Film wrapper	Covering, protecting containers	
Shrink seal	Stretch group of containers	
Bottle mouth seal	Tamper seal bottle containers	

Tape seal	Covering the cap of container	
Breakable seal	Opening evident	
Sealed tubes	Protecting the product and security seal	
Foil, paper, plastic pouches	Containing dose and different solid products	
Aerosol containers	Contains pressurized spray aerosol seal	
Sealed carton	Covering and protecting carton	

1.7.11 Child Proof Containers:

Child resistant containers CR may be either single-or two-pieces design. They require two or more motions to open making removal by a child is difficult. The most common motions are press and turn or squeeze and lock.

Figure 1-19 child-proof containers

The Latest in Child-Resistant...

1.7.12 Some Toxic Effects of Leachable Substances:

PVC leaches the plasticizer diethylhexylphthalate into drug solution containing lipid, surfactant or cosolvent. It is human carcinogenic.

Nitroglycerin should be packed in glass container because of adsorption on plastic and rubber.

Rubber stopper and syringe plunger can leach metal, 2-mercaptobezothiazole and nitroamines.

1.7.13 Comparison of Packaging Material Based on the Pack Requirements:

Property	Glass	Metal	Plastic
Weight	Heavy	Light	Light
Compatibility to product	Inert	React with the content, surface should be coated	Varies with the nature of the plastic.
Permeability to gas, vapor, odor	Impermeable	Excellent barrier	Depends on its nature
Stability at high temperature	Stable	Stable	Sensitive
Clarity / opacity	Clear	Opaque not clear.	Can be clear or opaque
Strength	Strong	Strong	Depends on its nature & density
Shatterproof	Breakable	Yes	Yes
Recycle	Yes	Yes	Easily recyclable
Cost	High	Less than glass	Cheep

1.7.14 Leaching, Adsorption, Permeability and Sterilization of Different Packaging Material:

Material	Leaching Leach extend		Adsorp extend	Permeability Water gases		sterilization
Borosilicate glass	Alkali metal oxides	1	2	0	0	Autoclave / dry heat
Sodalime glass	Metal oxides	5	2	0	0	Dry heat
HDPE	Antioxidant	1	2	3	3	Radiation / EO
LDPE	Plasticizer/ antioxidant	2	2	5	5	Radiation/ EO
PVC	Plasticizer/ stabilizer	4	2	5	2	Radiation / EO
PP	Antioxidant/ lubricant	2	1	5	3	Radiation / EO
Rubber natural	Metal salts/ lubricant	3	2	1	1	Autoclave / radiation
Rubber butyl	Metal salts/ lubricant	3	2	1	1	Autoclave /radiation
Rubber	Minimal	2	1	5	5	Autoclave /radiation

Section 2:

Quality Assurance for Packaging

2. Quality Assurance Packaging Index

no	Title
2.1	Sampling for testing packaging
2.2	Quality assurance for packaging
2.2.2	Packing design
2.2.3	Packaging specification
2.2.4	Qualification of suppliers
2.2.5	Quality parameters
2.2.5.1	Dimensions and measurements
2.2.5.2	Performance testing
2.2.5.3	Defects evaluation
2.2.6	Packaging evaluation and qualification
2.2.6.1	Validation of Packaging
2.2.6.2	Qualification of Packaging
2.2.6.3	Inspection of Packaging
2.2.6.4	Transport evaluation
2.2.7	Flexible packaging
2.2.8	USFDA requirements for packaging
2.2.9	Influence of stability testing on packaging

2.1 Sampling

Sampling is used to:

1- Check the correctness of the label, packaging material or containers.

2- To detect any countified medicines.

3- To retain samples to check stability, quality and shelf life.

4- To detect homogeneity, consistency and uniformity of material.

5- To represent the entire population.

Samples should be documented and according to SOPs.

2.1.1 Factors Governing the Sampling Process

1- Speed of machine; high speed packing machine requires larger sample size than hand packing.

2- New supplier; larger sample size is required for new supplier that that from a well-established one.

3- Sterile / clean components; testing sterile or clean components requires excessive procedures and either of the following measures may be followed:

   → Visit the supplier and obtain samples.

   → Predelivery of samples from the supplier.

   → Adopting supplier QC results after site inspection.

   → Having a special sterile facility for testing.

4- Reel fed laminates; it can be examined at the reel beginning or the supplier may provide samples from several points before slitting and validate and certify this process.

2.1.2 Sample Size for Batches:

Batch size	Sample size
3,201–10,000	200
10,001–35,000	315
35,001–150,000	500

2.1.3 SOPs for Sampling and Checking

1- Review supplier documents.

2- Review the container labeling.

3- Identify container type, size and integrity.

4- Inspect the container, pellets and stacking.

5- Record any observed defects.

Errors in any labelling, printing issues and errors or mistakes in the inserts or breakage/ damage of the container may be critical factors that may lead to rejection of consignments.

2.2 Quality Assurance for Packaging

Quality assurance for packaging is one of the components of GMP which involves the concern with designing the packaging component, its suitability to the product, its compatibility with the production machinery lines and its convenience to the market and users. The convenience to the market requires a constructed survey to investigate the market needs. In one company survey, it had been found that the major problem leading to the low level of sales is the poor packaging design and faint colours used. After changing the design and colours, significant improvement of sale was achieved.

However, quality assurance of packaging includes all aspects of design, specifications, supplier and quality performance parameters as well as validation of process and qualification of machineries. The same as other GMP components, it follows international specifications and inspection as well as waste disposal and evaluation of transport, handling and shipment.

Sampling and quality control procedures are the major subjects in quality assurance program.

2.2.1 Manifestations of Packaging Deficiencies

- x Breakage or damage.

- x Printing faults.

- x Ink errors.

- x Label information miss leading.

- x Adhesive ability dis-functioning.

- x Insert mistakes.

All of these simple defects can lead to product recall and results in drastic consequences but following GMP parameters and procedures minimizes facing such problems.

Validation of the packaging process and qualification of the machineries are facets of the GMP requirements.

2.2.2 Packaging Design

Unlike cosmetics, the design for pharmaceuticals should follow ethical medical parameters.

An ideal pack is the functional one that it is suitable for the product, protecting it throughout its shelf life without affecting its stability and that is complying the national drug authority regulations and guidelines.

Elements of good design

Design finalization

On design finalization a mock design simulating the final design should be made and trials assessment should be carried out including:

- ✓ Tooling and samples.

- ✓ Machine trials.

- ✓ Laboratory testing.

- ✓ Field trials.

Then modification if required and retrial, then validation of the process and lastly approval of drawings, documented and considered as specifications.

2.2.3 Packaging Specifications

For each design a final document is set as specifications and for each material there should be a document of the approved quality and tests for the standard specifications and a reference acceptable quality level AQL.

2.2.3.1 Stability Parameters

The specifications should provide a protective barrier for the product to maintain its potency throughout its shelf life without affecting its stability. This requires:

a- Moisture, vapor and gas protection.

b- Light barrier.

c- Temperature product as possible.

d- Should not alter the pH.

e- Should protect the contents against microbial contamination; neither ingression from the outside the container nor proliferation of included microbial limit.

2.2.3.2 Compatibility parameters

a- There should be no migration of ingredients such as preservatives and volatile substances from the drug to the packaging material.

b- There should be no leachable of materials such as stabilizers, plasticizer, antioxidant, slip additives and particulate from the packaging to the drug.

2.2.3.3 Physical attributes in setting specifications

a- Component dimensions.

b- Reliability of machine speed.

c- Scheduling of batches, stock policy, batch size and cost.

d- Capabilities of distribution channels.

e- Legislations concerning labelling, storage and fill weight.

f- Supplier ability and requirements.

g- Aesthetic considerations regarding the market policy and product classification.

2.2.3.4 Specifications given by regulatory authorities

a- BS 795: 1983 for ampoules.

b- BS 2006: 1984 for aluminum collapsible tubes.

c- BS 5597: 1991 for plastic aerosol containers.

d- BS 6652: 1985 for child resistant closure.

e- EN 293622:1983 for rubber closure for injectables.

2.2.4 Qualification of Supplier and Supplier Audit

The objectives of supplier qualification and auditing are:

a- To prevent defects at source.

b- To construct with the supplier the compliance certificate.

c- To monitor the production of the components to build confidence and reliance.

d- To assess the supplier manufacturing facility and confirm whether it can satisfy the requirements of quality and to assess whether the production capacity can fulfil the required quantities.

Auditing of the GMP dimensions of documentation, records, In-process control IPC, SOPs together with the batch release procedures give a clear picture of the supplier profile.

The supplier should have a contractual adherence to the specifications, QC tests and the manufacturing procedures of acceptance and rejection of consignments. This will build a long bilateral benefit relationship. The specification of each material should include QC testing and extend of routine testing. The program depends on the policy and standards, the level of confidence, the manufacturing capacity and the market requirements. Continuous improvement could be achieved through total quality management TQM, Just-in-time JIT, Statistical Process Control SPC to minimize the variability, improve consistency and reduce the cost.

2.2.5 Quality Parameters

The quality tests include:

1- Identification of material

2- Visual inspection; cleanness and defects.

3- Dimensional measurements.

4- Physical tests.

5- Chemical tests.

6- Microbiological tests.

7- Quantification.

8- Functional and performance tests.

9- Defect classification.

10- Action plan and records.

A. **Identification**

Description against the standards and recognizing the batch number.

Quantity grammage; grammage of paper, foils, films and laminates.

B. <u>Visual inspection</u>

Visual inspection by well-trained technician to check the printed text and match the colours against the specifications and artwork and notify the defects, table 2-1.

Table 2-1 Visual inspection for packaging

Material	Examination
Labels, cartons, leaflet	Test accuracy, legibility, trimming, construction mistakes, adhesive failure, contamination.
Plastic containers	Molding, sink marks, flash and thin spots.
Glass containers	Splits, checks, chips, strains & contamination.
Vials & ampoules	Glass particulate.
Reel laminates	Slackly wound, incorrect winding direction.

Visual inspection includes any mix-up or adulteration by by other designs or other batches. It also includes the pack of container, stacking, damage, labelling and presentation.

2.2.5.1 Dimensions and measurements

The following table is the measurements that should be taken for some packaging components.

Table 2-2 Dimensions and measurements

Component	Measurements
Ampoules	Height/outer diameter/constriction outer diameter
Vials	Height/outer diameter/finish profile.
Plastic bottle	Major-minor outer diameter, wall thickness, finishing.
Rubber stopper	Height, outer diameter, flange thickness.

<u>Measuring tools:</u>

Gauge, calipers, optical devices and computer-link equipment can be used as a measuring tool.

2.2.5.2 Performance and functional tests

These tests include the followings:

a- Capacity of bottle, vials and ampoules.

b- Hardness of rubber.

c- Heat seal strength of laminate, films and labels.

d- Multicomponent assembly for containers, closures and devices.

e- Leakage and spray patterns.

2.2.5.3 Defect evaluation

The classification of defects depends on it effects to the patient, to the product and to the production process. These defects are categorized into four categories with respect to the Acceptance Quality Level AQL.

Table 2-3 Classification of defects

Category	AQL	Effect	Description
	2.5-4%	Minor	Non-functional, slight visual fault. Noticeable by user.
	0.65-1.5%	Major	Substandard performance, visually objectionable.
	0.1-0.4%	Critical	Adversely affect the performance of product or packaging.
	0%	Intolerable	Accept 0, reject one as in case of mix-up.

2.2.6 Validation and Qualification of Packaging

2.2.6.1 Validation of packaging

The packaging validation includes:

a- Design validation;

To confirm whether the specifications conforms with the user needs and the intended use.

b- The packaging process validation;

To provide an evidence that the process consistently produces a product complying the predetermined specifications.

2.2.6.2 Qualification of packaging

based on the dosage form and route of administration are information that should be provided to proof that the container-closure system is suitable for its intended use. Qualification requires performing the following tests:

a- Protection from light: The light transmission test using spectrophotometer to measure the amount of light transmitted by the plastic material of the container.

b- Protection against water vapor is tested by water vapor permeation test USP <661> limits.

c- Protection against ingression can be tested by dye or microbial ingression test and quantified using helium photometry.

d- Compatibility: this test requires test for leachables at intervals throughout the product shelf life using chemical detection and quantification techniques.

e- Safety: the physiochemical tests for water soluble plastic extractables are performed to determine their biological reactivity to specify the safety level of exposure.

f- Performance: this attribute is to test the functionality towards the patient compliance, minimizing the waste and ease of use. It considered the drug delivery, the required amount of the prescribed dose at the required rate. This test considers the pre-filled syringes, transdermal patches, MDI and spray containers.

2.2.6.3 Inspection of packaging

Inspection should be carried out by an expert, well trained technician. It should be fast and use electronic device whenever it is possible.

Caliper, gauges, optical operators and computer-link devices whenever they are available. Weight can be checked automatically, machine vision system can test the volume and scanning the label. Metal detection can be detected by X-ray devices. Helium leak can rapidly detect the leakage.

2.2.6.4 Evaluation of Transport

Packaging are subjected to various factors during transportation.

a- Mechanical stress and staking pressure.

b- Climatic conditions.

c- Vibration, dropping and shock during handling and transportation.

The transport evaluation can be carried out by the following tests:

1- Compression strength testing by subjecting the package to compression force and evaluate the force that it can tolerate.

2- Distribution simulation test: this is to test the ability of the packaging to withstand the distribution handling and storage compression.

2.2.7 Flexible Packaging

Blister for packaging of tablets and capsules.

   Sachets for packaging of powder and unit dose.

Flexible packaging includes plastic bags, foil liding, blister and strip packaging, foil bags and sachets.

Materials are polyethylene, polypropylene, polyester or polyurethane and laminates. Blister packaging consists of aluminum foil is the lidding layer at the base side which is usually printed and a forming film a heat-sealing lacquer on the other side. The pouch is usually sealed at the three sides leaving the upper side open for filling.

Most common flexible materials are:

Aluminum foil, biaxial oriented polypropylene, Low density polyethylene, linear low-density polyethylene, oriented poly propylene OPP, polyamide, PE, polyethylene phthalate, polyvinylchloride PVC and polyvinylidene chloride PVDC.

2.2.8 US FDA Requirements

1- Primary packaging materials should be manufacture in class C clean room.

2- The container should pass physical teats <661> USP.

3- It should not be composed of any hazardous compound.

4- It should provide protection to the contents from the surrounding environment throughout content shelf life.

5- It should not react, sorb or add any substances beyond the established limits.

6- It should not alter the purity, strength or efficacy of the drug.

7- The flexible material should maintain its integrity throughout the shelf life of the product.

8- Recycled material should not be used.

9- The material should have CoA and CoC from the supplier whom should be audited periodically.

10- CoA and CoC should include data that complies the manufacture acceptance criteria.

11- Drawing and dimensions should be provided.

12- Complete process description and process validation, QC tests for various attributes should be provided.

13- The following tests should be performed:

    a- Multiple internal reflectance for HDPE and LDPE.

    b- Light transmission.

    c- Water vapor permeation.

    d- Heavy metal.

    e- Non-volatile residue.

2.2.9 Influence of Stability Testing Conditions on the Packaging

Packaging materials may withstand stability testing condition of long-term stability testing and accelerated stability testing for the specified period but fail to withstand cycling or stress conditions stability testing.

Packaging may be influenced by higher temperature and relative humidity, vibration, compression and pH changes.

When a semipermeable container exposed to higher or lower humidity, it may lead to alternation or changes in the stability of the product.

Closure efficiency may be changed in various storage conditions. Changes before, during and after packaging should be checked by expert technician to identify the integrity, uniformity, safety and effectiveness of material in such an economically acceptable art.

Section 3:

Quality Control tests for Packaging

3.1 Quality Control Tests Overview

Quality control tests is performed for the following packaging components:

☞ Glass container.

☞ Plastic container.

☞ Closures.

☞ Collapsible tubes.

☞ Metallic tin containers.

☞ Strips and blisters.

☞ Cartons.

☞ Paper and board.

The tests to be carried out at reputable and reliable laboratory following Good Laboratory Practice and being licensed by the regulatory authority.

The tests to be performed are summarized at table 3-1 for glass containers, plastic containers and closures. Collapsible tubes, metallic tin, blister and strips, carton and paper and board are mentioned.

Table 3-1 Summary of the test to be carried out

	Glass containers	Plastic containers	Closures
1	Chemical resistance - powdered glass - water attack	Collapsibility test	Sterility
2	Hydraulic resistance	Leakage test	Penetrability
3	Thermal shock	Clarity test	Fragmentation
4	Internal bursting pressure	Non-volatile residue	Self-sealability
5	Leakage test	Water permeability	pH of aqueous extract
6	Arsenic test	Transparency	Residue on evaporation
7	Annealing test	Acidity or alkalinity	Light absorbance
8	Vertical load test	Reducing substances	Reducing substances
9	Autoclaving test	Biological activity	

Collapsible tubes	Metallic tin	Blister/ strip	Cartons	Paper & board
-leakage test	Description	Leakage test	Compression	Refer to text
Lacquer curing	Dimensions		Opening orifice	
Lacquer compatibility	Diameter		Coefficient of friction	
	cleanliness		Crease stiffness	
			Joint shear strength	

3.2 Quality Control Tests for Glass Containers

3.2.1 Chemical Resistance of Glass Container

a. Powdered glass test

This test is performed to determine the amount of alkali leached from glass which enhanced by elevated temperature. It is an acid-base titration using 0.02 N H_2So_4 and methyl red as an indicator. USP specifies the volume according to glass type <660>.

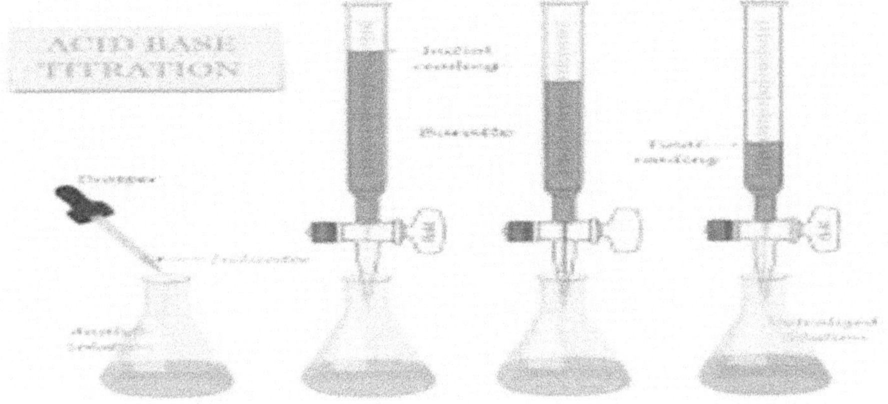

Figure 3-1 Acid-base titration process

preparing the speciemen

- few containers rinsed throughly with purified water, dried with clean steam.
- triturate in a mortor to fine powder and pass through sevie 20 and 50.

washing the specimen

- 10 gms is placed in 250 ml conical flask and washed with 30 ml acetone.
- repeat the washing and decant acetone, dry it and use the specimen within 4 hours.

procedure

- 10 gms in 250 ml conical flask, add 50 ml highly pirified water, place in an autoclave at 121 °C for 30 min then cool under running water.
- decant the solution into another flask, wash with 15 ml highly purified water and again decant.
- titrate immediately with 0.02 N H_2So_4 using methyl red as an indicator and record the volume.

b. Water attack test

This test is carried out for treated sola lime glass to assess the leaching of alkali from the inner treated surface of the container.

→ Rinse thoroughly 3 or more containers with highly purified water.

→ Fill each container to 90% of it over flow capacity with highly purified water.

→ Cap the flasks and autoclave at 121 °C for 60 min.

→ Cool and decant into 250 ml conical flask to volume of 100 ml.

→ Add 3 drops of methyl red solution.

→ Titrate with 0.02N H2So4.

→ Record the volume of sulphuric acid.

⁂ This is a measure for the amount of alkaline oxides present in the surface of glass container.

Figure 3-2: Titration

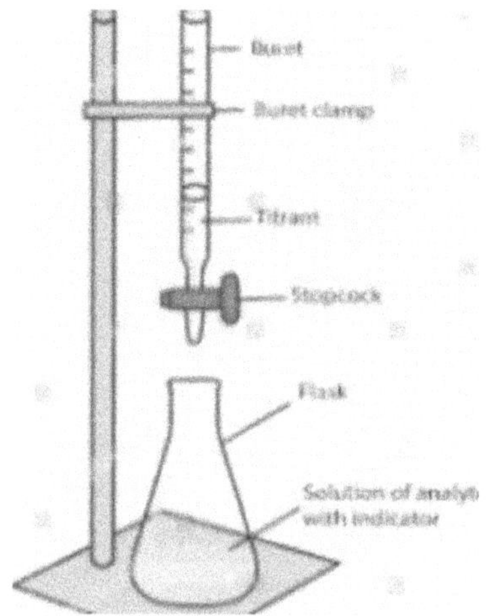

Table 3-2 Test limits

Test	Container	Volume of 0.02N H_2So_4
Powder glass test	Type I	1
	Type II	8.5
	Type III	15
Water attack	Type II 100 ml or below	0.7
	Type II above 100 ml	0.2

3.2.2 Hydraulic Resistance of Glass Containers

Table 3-3 Number of containers and volume of solution to be used:

Nomonal capacity	Number of containers	Volume of test solution to be used for titration
5 ml or less	At least 10	50 ml
6 ml – 30 ml	At least 5	50 ml
More than 30 ml	At least 3	1000 ml

<u>**Procedure:**</u>

⧗ Take the number of containers as per the table above.

→ Rinse each container at least 3 times with distilled water.

→ Fill with distilled water to the filling volume.

→ Heat to 100 °C for 10 min and allow the steam to flow from the vent cork.

→ Raise the temperature to 121°C in 20 min and maintain it for 60 min.

→ Lower the temperature to 100 °C for 40 min with venting to prevent vacuum.

→ Remove the containers from the autoclave and cool.

→ Combine the liquid to examined.

→ Measure the volume of test solution into conical flask.

→ Titrate with 0.01 M HCl using methyl red as an indicator.

→ Perform blank using water.

✓ The difference between titrations represents the volume of 0.01 M HCl consumed by the test solution.

✓ The specified volume is given in the table 3-4.

Table 3-4 Volume of acid corresponding to container volume

Capacity of container corresponding 90% over flow volume (ml)	Volume of 0.01M HCl per 100 ml test solution	
	Type I & type II glass ml	Type III glass ml
Not more than I ml	2	20
More than 1 ml but not more than 2 ml	1.8	17.6
More than 2 ml but not more than 5 ml	1.3	13.2
More than 5 ml but not more than 10 ml	1	10.2
More than 10 ml but not more than 20 ml	0.8	8.1
More than 20 ml but not more than 50 ml	0.6	6.1
More than 50 ml but not more than 100 ml	0.5	4.8
More than 100 ml but not more than 200 ml	0.4	3.8
More than 200 ml but not more than 500 ml	0.3	2.9
More than 500 ml	0.2	2.2

3.2.3 Thermal Shock Test

→ Place the samples in an upright position in a tray.

→ Immerse the tray in a hot water for a given time.

→ Transfer to a cold-water bath of 45 °C difference from the hot water.

→ Examine the cracks or breaks before and after the test figure 3-4.

→ The thermal shock a bottle can afford depends on its size, design and glass distribution. Small bottles afford differential 60 – 80°C and I pint bottle can afford differential of 30 – 40°C.

Figure 3-3 Thermal shock cracks
[g araboglass.com – Guangzhou]

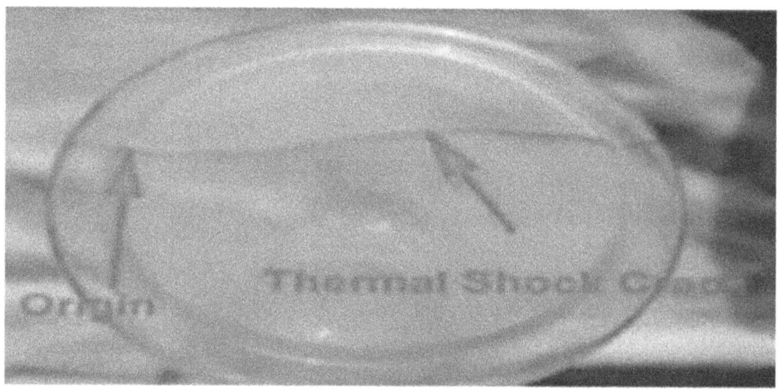

3.2.4 Internal Bursting Pressure Test

The American glass research increment pressure tester is the commonly used instrument for this test.

→ The bottle is filled with water and placed in the test chamber, a scale head is applied and the internal pressure automatically and gradually increased by a series of increments. Each increment is maintained for a given time.

→ At each preselected level, the tested bottle is checked until the pressure at which the bottle bursts. This is the resulting end point.

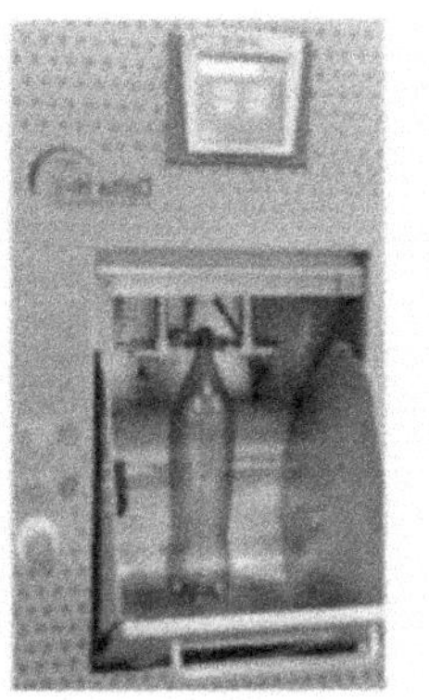 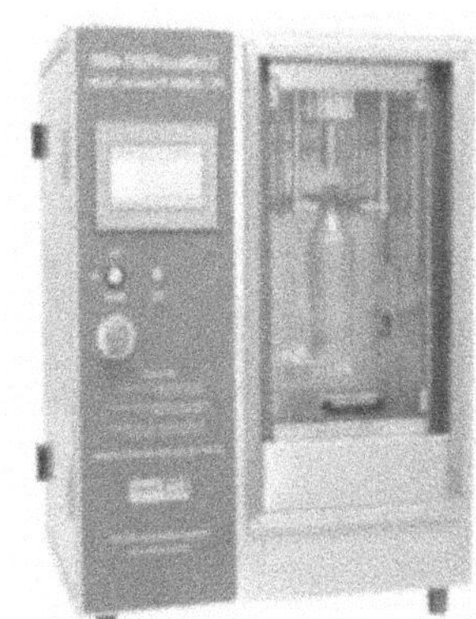 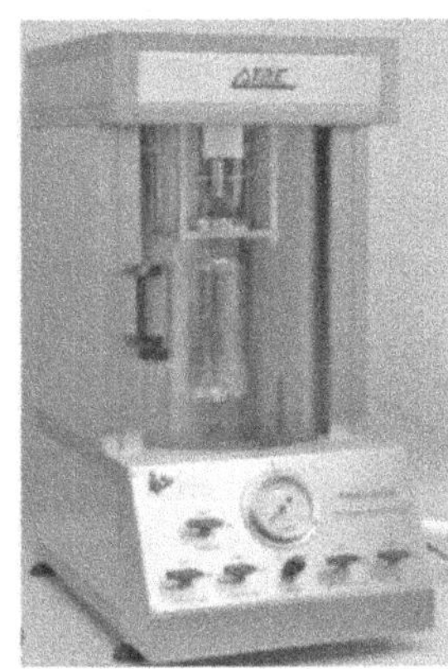

Figures 3-4, 3-5: Internal pressure burst tester.
[1-Farmakim Laboratuvar, Turkey. 2-IDM-Instrument,
Australia. 3-atze-usa.com]

3.2.5 Leakage Test

fill 10 containers with water and fit the intended closure.

keep them inverted for 24 hours at room temperature

the test is said to be passed if no signs of leakage of any container.

Alternatively: the filled containers can be placed in a coloured solution and vacuum is applied and check if the colour entered the container.

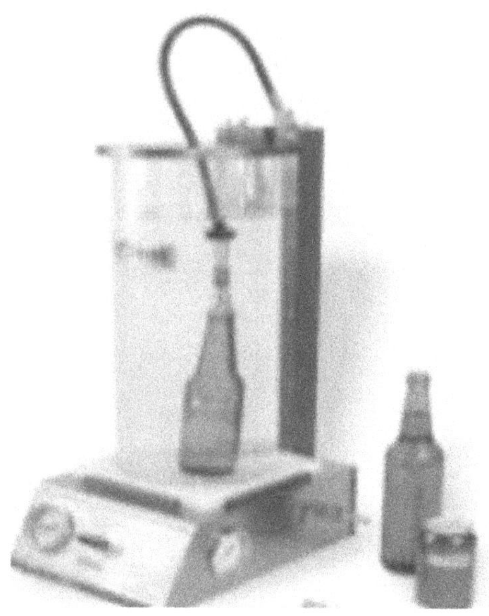

3-6 Leakage tester [Effective lab, India-Indian mart]

3.2.6 Arsenic Test

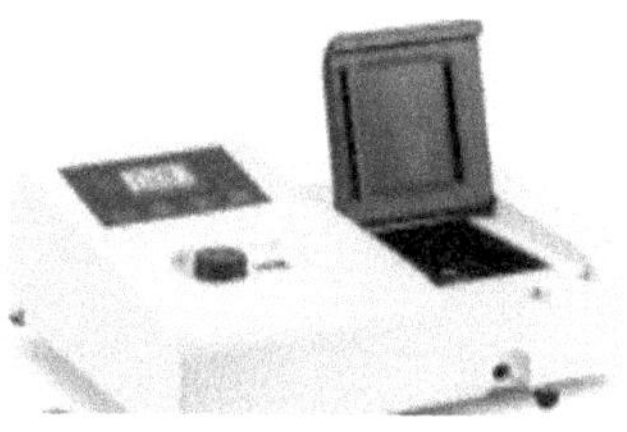

This test is performed for glass containers intended to be used for aqueous parenteral solutions.

→ Use enough number of containers.

→ Wash the inner and outer by distilled water for 5 minutes.

→ Fill with distilled water, heat to 100 °C for 10 min and dry by clean steam.

→ Rise the temperature to 121°C for 20 mins and maintain it for 60 mins, then lower the temperature to 100°C and remove from the autoclave.

→ Combine the liquid to obtain 50 ml.

→ Add 10 ml HNO3, dry on water bath then in oven at 130°C for 30 mins and let to cool.

→ Add 10 ml hydrogen molybdate, swirl to dissolve and heat on water bath for 25 mins.

→ Cool to room temperature.

→ Measure the absorbance at 840 nm.

→ The absorbance should not exceed that of a solution of 0.1 ml arsenic standard solution (NMT 10 ppm).

3.2.7 Annealing Test

The sample is examined by polarized light and compared with a standard disc.

3.2.8 Vertical Load Test

The bottle is placed between a vertical plarform and hydraulic ramp placed to provide vertical compression on the bottle. The hydraulic ram is raised gradually and the load is recorded by pressure gauge.

Figure 3-7 Vertical load tester

[Agr International Inc, agrint.com]

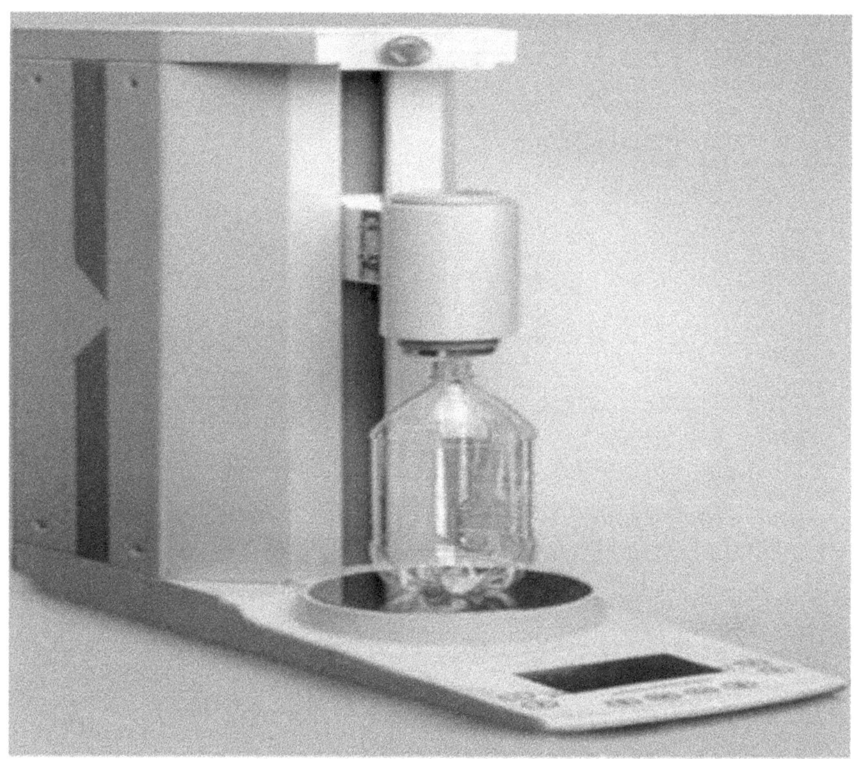

3.2.9 Autoclaving Test

Checking the ability of empty and filled container s to withstand autoclaving at 121 °C for 60 minutes.

Figure 3-8 Autoclaves

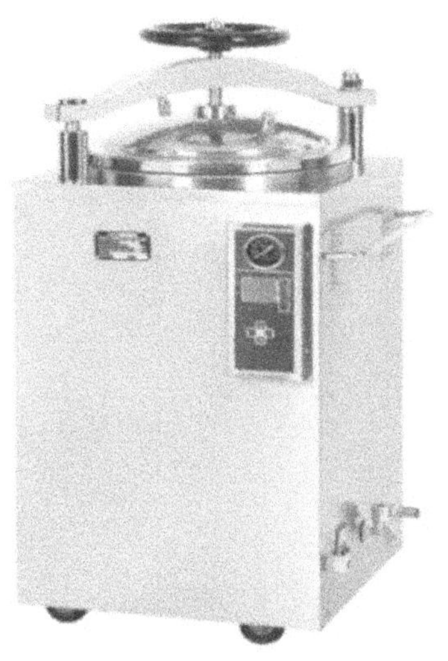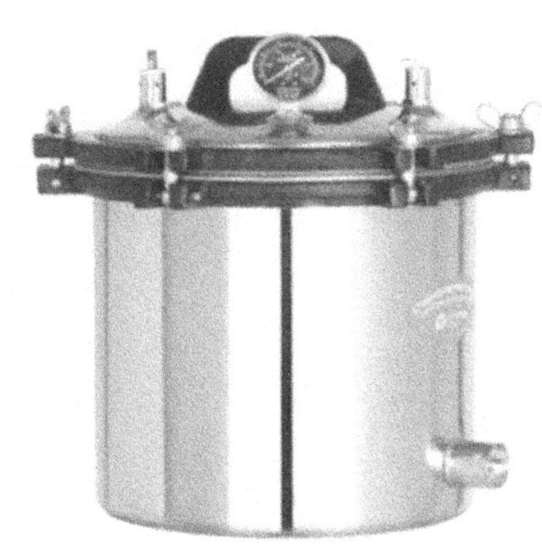

3.3 Quality Control Tests for Plastic Containers

The followings are the tests to be carried out for plastic containers:

Collapsibility test	*Acidity & alkalinity test*	*Non-volatile residue test*
Leakage test	*Clarity test*	*Reducing substance test*
Permeability test	*Transparency test*	*Biological tests.*

3.3.1 Collapsibility Test

This test is for containers that to be squeezed to deliver their content. The container should release 90% of its content at specified flow rate at ambient temperature upon inward collapsing.

Figure 3-9 Collapsibility tester may be used.

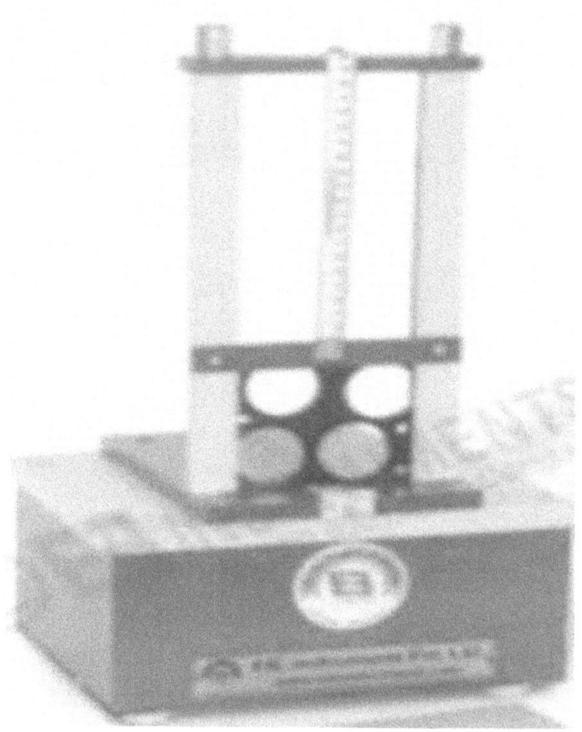

3.3.2 Leakage Test

This test is performed for plastic containers using traditional method of filling 10 containers with water, closed, then inverted and kept for 24 hours. Check the leak or wetting of the area.

Recent technologies used leakage tester which uses positive and negative pressure procedures. The bottles are used empty, surrounded by a water in a chamber, then apply positive pressure and check the presence of water inside the bottle. The other method is to fill the bottle in a dry chamber and then apply a negative pressure and check the scape of water outside the bottle.

Figure 3-10 leakage testing

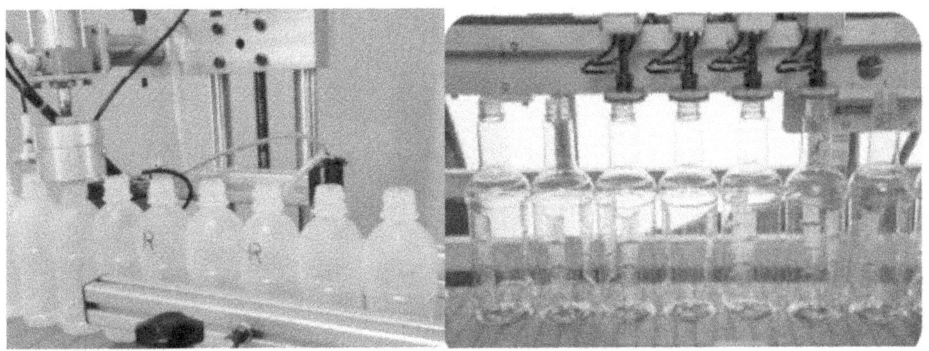

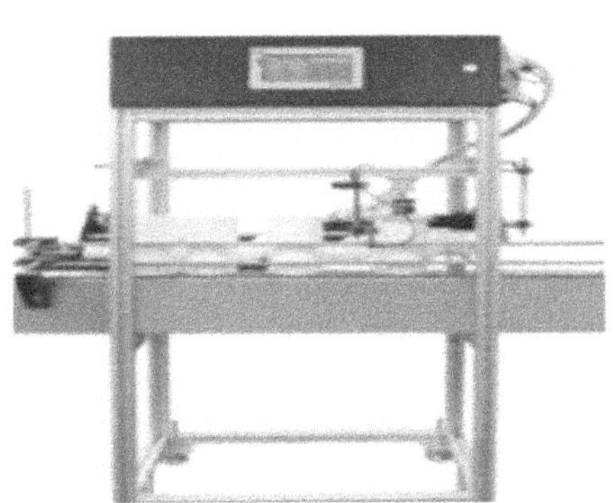

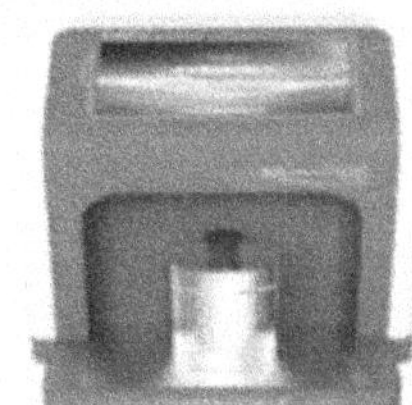

3.3.3 Water Permeability Test

→ Fill 5 containers with water to their nominal volume, heat-seal the bottles or closed with aluminum foil and weigh each bottle.

→ Allow to stand for 14 days at 20-25°C/ 60% RH.

→ Reweigh the containers.

- The loss in weight in each container NMT 0.2%.

3.3.4 Clarity Test

Preparation of clarity solution:

→ Strips are taken from a well cleaned containers of area NMT 20 cm². Wash twice with distilled water for 30 minutes then placed into a clean flask.

→ Prepare a blank.

→ Autoclave both flasks at 121°C for 30minutes and cool.

→ Compare the tested sample and the blank.

✓ There should be no any sort of turbidity

✓ Using light absorbance at 230-360 nm the difference of test from the blank should be NMT 0.2.

3.3.5 Transparency Test

→ Prepare a standard suspension of 1:200 from PP or PE containers.

→ Fill the containers with this suspension to their nominal volume.

✓ The cloudiness of the suspension is perceptible when viewed through the container and compared with other container filled with water.

3.3.6 Acidity and Alkalinity

From the solution obtain in the clarity test, take 4%of the container capacity and add 0.1 ml phenolphethaline solution., the solution is colorless.

→ Add 0.4 ml of 0.01 M NaOH, the solution is pink.

→ Add 0.01 M HCl and 0.1 methyl red, the solution is orange-red.

3.3.7 Non-Volatile Residue Test

From the extract obtained in the clarity test, take 100 ml and dry it at 105°C until a constant weight is obtained.

✓ The residue weight should be NMT 12.5 mg.

3.3.8 Reducing Substances

- From the solution obtained from the clarity test, take 20 ml and add 1 ml dilute H_2SO_4 and 20 ml of 0.002M $KMnO_4$.

→ Boil for 3 mins and cool.

→ Add 1 gm KI and titrate immediately with 0.01 M Na_2SO_3 using 0.25 ml of starch solution as indicator.

→ Titrate using blank test proceeded in the same way.

→ The difference between 0.01 M sodium thiosulphate volumes is NMT 1.5 ml.

3.3.9 Biological Tests

A- A group of 5 Albino mice is injected by the test solution and observed at times:

Zero, 4hrs, 24 hrs, 48 hrs and 72 hrs.

→ Another group of 5 mice is injected with blank on the same way as a control group.

→ Observe the two groups together.

✓ The test is passed if no significant reactivity in all of the groups.

- If convulsions, prostration or more than 2 grams body loss is observed, the sample failed the test.

B- Intracutaneously inject a rabbit by the test solution and check the reaction like erythema, edema and necrosis at 24, 48 and 72 hours.

The difference between test and blank scores is less than 1.

C- Eye irritation test:

Drops of the sample extract are applied to the rabbit eye, there should be no significant irritation response compared with a blank.

3.4 Quality Control Tests for Closures

<u>Preparation of the sample solution (solution A)</u>

Using anionic surfactant 0.2% W/V wash the sample 5 times. Rinse 5 times with distilled water, add 200 ml water and autoclave at 121°C for 20-30 minutes. Cover with Aluminum foil and let to cool. Then decant the solution. Use this solution as solution A.

3.4.1 Sterility Test

Closures are subjected to sterility tested using the specified sterile media at 65°C and pressure of 0.7 Kpar for 24 hours.

3.4.2 Penetrability Test

The rubber closure should let the needle to pass through it by pressing force not more than 10 N. the needle should not bent or damaged by the excessive force. This force can be measured by Penetrability tester.

Figure 3-11 Permeability Tester *[Mecmesin.com – UK]*

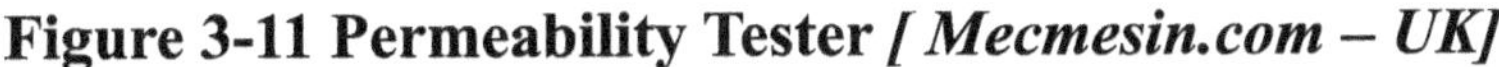

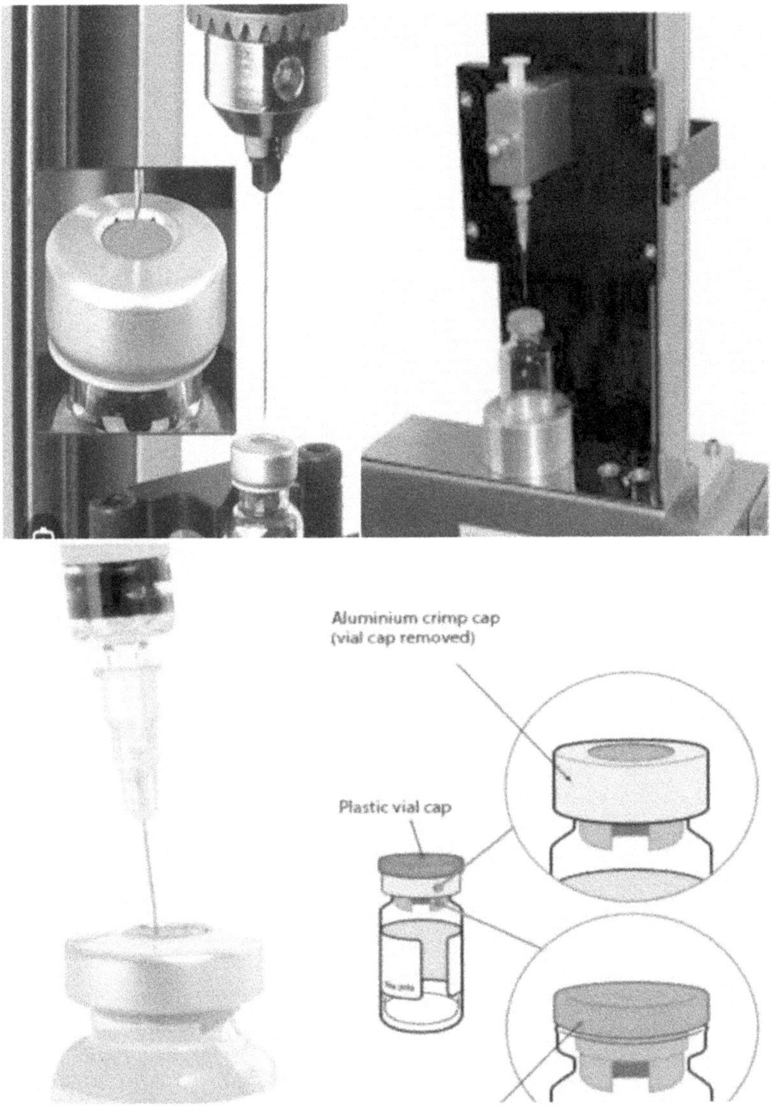

3.4.3 Fragmentation Test

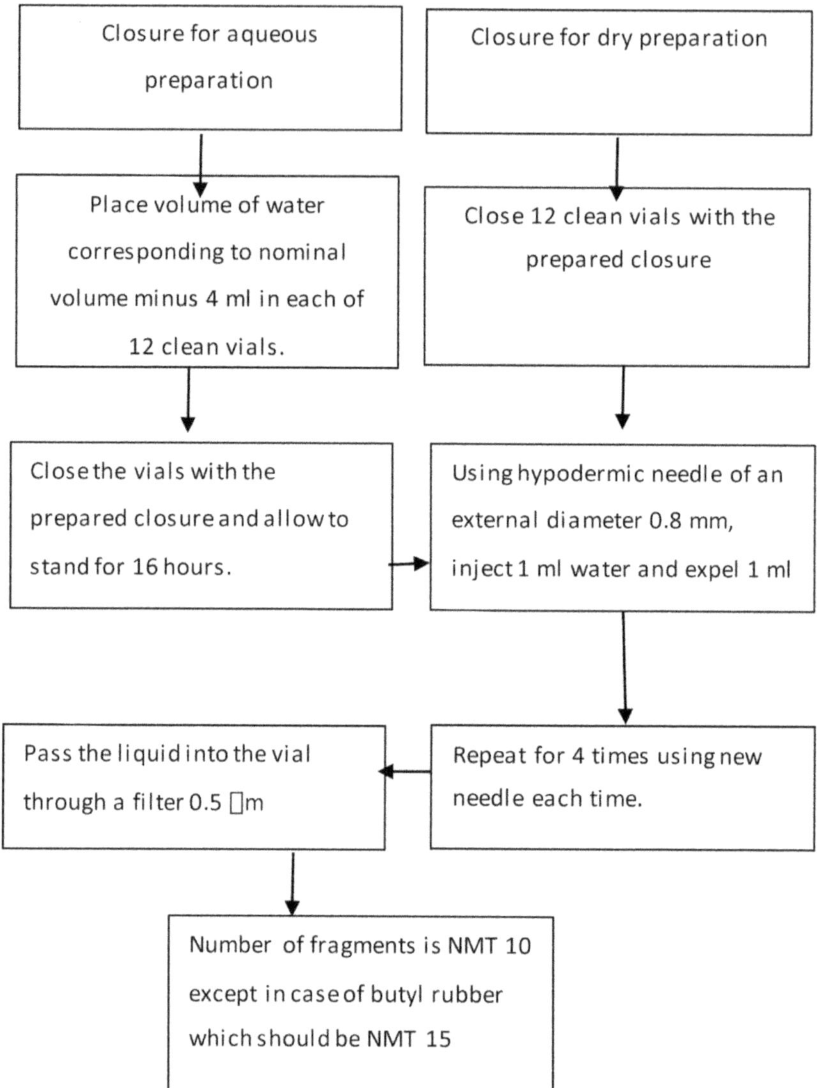

3.4.4 Self-Sealability Test

For each closure, use a new hypodermic needle of an external diameter 0.8 mm and pierce the closure 10 times. Each time at a different site.

- → Immerse the vail in an upright position in a 0.1% w/v methylene blue solution and reduce the external pressure by 27 kpa for 10 minutes.

- → Restore the atmospheric pressure and leave vials immersed for 30 minutes.

- → Rinse the outer surface of vials.

  - ✓ None of the vials contains any traces of methylene blue solution.

3.4.5 pH of the Aqueous Extract

- take 20 ml of solution A + 0.1 ml bromothymol blue.

- Add 0.01 M NaOH, NMT 0.3 ml to change the colour to yellow.

- If using HCL, the volume of HCL needed to change the colour of bromothymol blue is NMT 0.8 ml.

3.4.6 Residue on Evaporation

- → Evaporate 50 ml of solution A to dryness at 105 °C

- ✓ The residue should not be more than 4 mg.

3.4.7 Light Absorbance Test

→ Use freshly prepared solution A to be used within 4 hours, filter through 0.5 mm and measure the absorbance at 220 – 360 nm.

3.4.8 Reducing Substances

→ 20 ml solution A + 1 ml H2SO4 + 0.002M KMnO4, boil for 3 min, cool and add 1ml KI. Titrate with Na2SO3 using starch as indicator.

→ Carry out a blank test.

✓ The difference between the two titrations should not be more than 0.7 ml.

3.5 Quality Control Tests for Collapsible Tubes

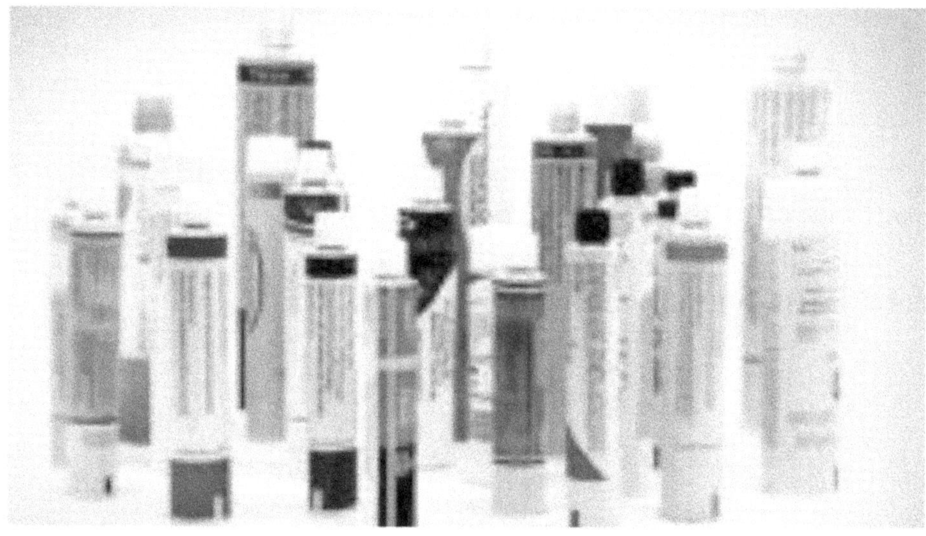

Figure 3-12 Examples of collapsible tubes

3.5.1 Leakage Test

A tube was filled with water, tightly closed and the surface is wiped off. Then, the tube is kept standing in an inverted position on a dry filter paper. After one hour the filter paper is checked whether it wetted or not or any water escape during the test.

3.5.2 Lacquer Curing Test

a- Adhesion force:

The tube was split longitudinally and flatted. Cotton wool soaked in acetone was used to rub over the lacquer surface for 20 minutes. Lacquer should not leave the surface and the cotton wool piece should stay uncoloured.

b- The tube was folded in such a way that the internal lacquer is to the outside, rubbed with finger, the lacquer should not be peeled off.

3.5.3 Lacquer Compatibility

→ 10 tubes were filled and crimped, subjected to 45 °C for 72 hours.

→ Cool and cut longitudinally.

✓ No discoloration or changes or gas formation in the content is observed.

✓ No lifting or peeling of the lacquer is observed.

3.5.4 Other Tests

1. The tube pantone colour.

2. Tube layers.

3. Tube thickness measurements.

4. Tube length measurements.

5. Tube diameter measurements.

6. Orifice measurements; length and diameter.

7. Screw cap opening power value.

8. Flip cap opening force value.

9. Tube sealing test.

10. Decorative peeling test.

11. Alcohol test.

12. Heating test.

Figure 3-13 Collapsibility tester

[altubecan.com, Yingrun machinery – Jiangsu, China]

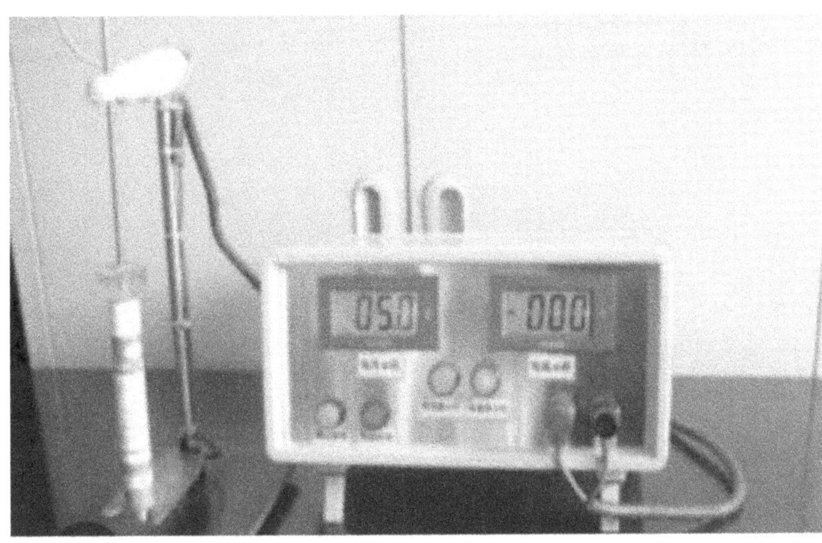

3.6 Quality Control Tests for Metallic Tin Containers

3.6.1 Description:

Description of the visual physical characteristics and the texture of the surface, the presence of seal and opening or cover specifications.

Figure 3-14 Examples of metallic containers

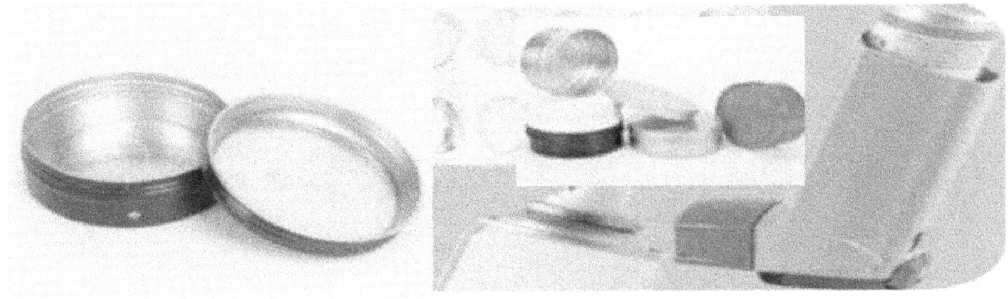

Dimensions

Height in mm: measure 10 tins, the limit tolerance is 170 mm ± 10 *mm*

Diameter

Inner diameter of tin tins, not less than 98 mm, the outer diameter limit NMT 105 mm.

Cleanness

It should be clean, free from dirt, damage, stain or any foreign material.

3.6.2 Microbiological Test for Tin Tubes

Process:

1
- 50 empty tubes, filled with ointment base and sealed.
- keep over night.

2
- a metal bacteriological filter fitted with filter paper.
- heated the metal to melting range of the ointment base.

3
- squeeze base from all tubes at a certain rate and pass through filter under vacuum.
- wash with $CHCl_3$ and examine presence of particles.

Observations

Table 3-5 Particle Size and Count

Particle size	Observed number
1 mm and above	50
0.5 – 1 mm	10
0.2 – 0.5 mm	2
Less than 0.2 mm	N/A
Total score	62

Limits

✓ Lot of tubes passed the test if the total score is less than 100.

x Lot of tubes failed the test if the total score is more than 150.

→ The test should be repeated again using 50 more tubes if the count is between 100 and 150.

3.7 Quality Control Tests for Strips and Blisters

Quality control tests for strips and blisters involves the following test:

1- The barrier properties.

2- The tensile strength.

3- The impact resistance strength.

4- The thermal tensile ratio.

5- The hygiene indexes.

Among all, the barrier test is the more important that it indicates the protection properties of the blister regarding gases and volatile substance to the inside and outside the blister.

It should guard the product from moisture and water vapour ingression.

The dye ingression test involves immersion of the blister in a solution of methylene blue in a desiccator and subject to vacuum of 200 – 600 mbar for several minutes.

Water on the outer surface is wiped off with a cotton wool, then the blister or strip is opened and check the content for the presence of water or dye.

→ No water or the content should not be wetted, this indicates no leakage and proper sealing.

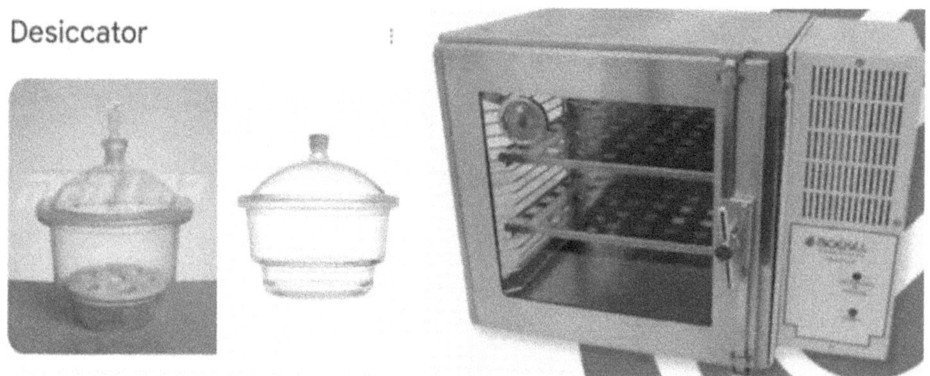

Figure 3-15 Desiccators *[Medlab-India]*

3.8 Quality Control Tests for Cartons

Table 3-6: Tests for cartons

Test	Uses
Compression	To assess the strength of erected package
Carton opening force	To hold the flat carton as delivered, by pressing its creases between thumb and first finger.
Coefficient of friction	Both static and kinetic coefficients of friction are determined by sliding the specimen over itself under the specified conditions.
Crease stiffness	Folding the carton on 90°. It will try to recover to its original state on removal of stress.
Joint shear strength	Testing the glued lap seam on the side of carton for strength of adhesion using a tensile strength machine.

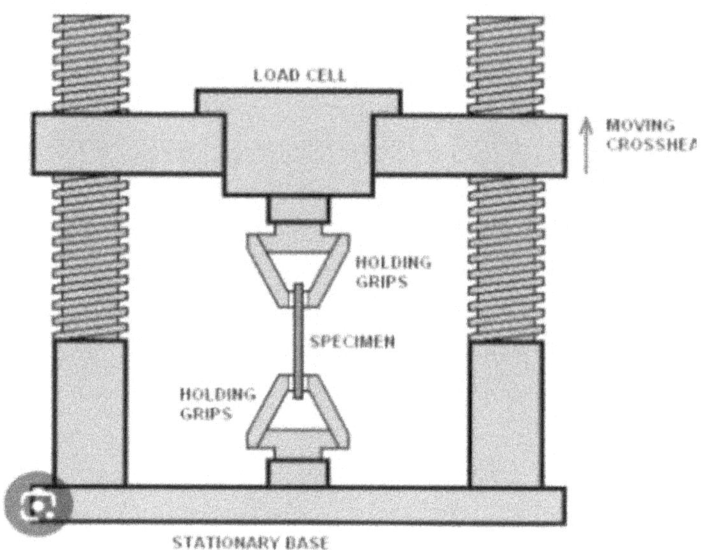

[Engineering Archives.2012]

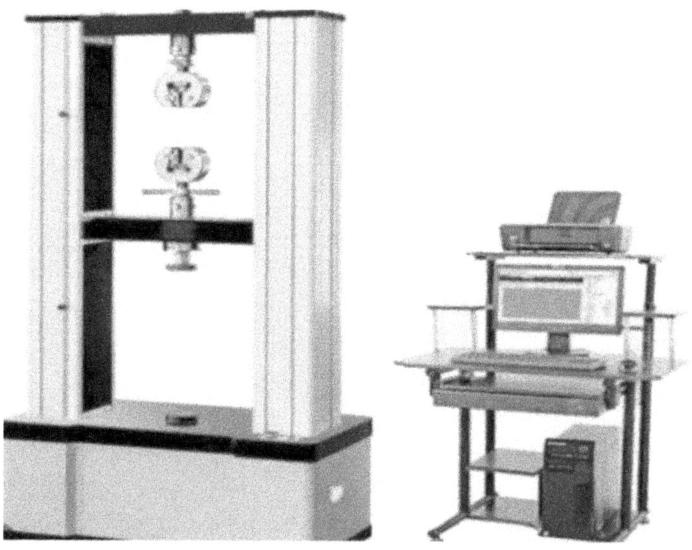

Figure 3-16 Tensile strength machine *[Labs NOVA-China]*

3.9 Quality Control Tests for Paper & Board

The following tests are carried out at 23 °C 1°C and relative humidity 50

Test	Description
Moisture content	Difference of two weights at specific conditions.
Folding durability	Fold the sample back and forth until rupture.
Density	For rigid cellular material.
Air permeability	For light weight uncoated paper on a machine using vacuum pick-up system. Expressed/pa/sec
Paper caliper	For the thickness of paper.
Tensile strength	Maximum tensile stress per unit width that a paper or board can withstand before breaking or permanently deformed.
Substance grammage	The weight of material/unit area; gm/m^2.
Burst strength	The maximum uniformly distributed pressure applied at 90° to the surface of the sample before it bursts. Hydraulic pressure is applied to diaphragm bulging it until it burst.
Tear strength	The mean force required to continue tearing of an initially cut in a single sheet of paper.
Puncture resistance	Energy required to make initial puncture.
Stiffness of thick paper and board	Degree of resistance of a sample when it is bent.

Creasibility of board	To determine quality of creasing of board within 300 – 100 μm.
Cobb test gm/m²	Test for water absorbance.
Rub resistance	Resistance of a printed sample to withstand rubbing against another similar one.
Pick test/IGT test	A specified oil is added to a printing system and printing on the sample. T hen examine the signs of pick.
pH, chloride or sulphate	The acidity and alkalinity can help the life of the paper board.
Roughness/smoothness	Essential for printing of paper.
Brightness	Reflectance factor measured at the effective range 457nm.
Ash test	To determine the ash content.
Wet burst strength	Bursting strength following immersion in water.
Wet tensile strength	Tensile strength on immersion in water.
Opacity	Percentage of luminous reflectance factor of a sheet black backed to the intrinsic luminous reflectance factor.
Detection and estimation of nitrogenous agents	Applied to dyes of strong affinity to acidic medium.
Ink absorbency	For determination of ink absorbency of paper or board by K & N ink.

Section 4:

Manufacturing of Single-use Plastic Syringes

4.1 Introduction

The disposable single use plastic syringes are devices composed of graduated cylindrical component known as the barrel and a plunger or piston moving inside the barrel to deliver the content which is usually fluid medicament. A stainless-steel needle is attached to the barrel at nozzle adapter. The needle pierces the skin without injury and deliver the medicine into the body tissue or blood stream through the hollow canal or sucking blood or fluid from the body.

The syringe is made of polypropylene or polyethylene pharmaceutical grade and the syringe is either to be filled before use or pre-filled syringe ready to be injected. They are sterile and of low cost, so it is a single use. The multi-use glass syringes use was increasingly decline because of the hazards of disease transmission like HIV, Hepatitis B and so one. The single use disposable syringes fill this gap and represents a durable cost-effective solution.

The disposable syringes are of many sizes and types, here we will consider the traditional 3 pieces syringes having the various sizes.

4.1.1 Common Sizes

1/ insulin disposable syringes of 1 ml or may be graduated in insulin units.

2/ 2ml, 2.5,3 ml, 5 ml, 10, 20,30 ml.

3/ large sizes for veterinary use and measuring tasks.

4/ Pre-filled syringes: according to the dose..

The syringes should be sterile and disposed after use, they can be used intramuscular, intravenous and subcutaneous.

Generally, sterilization by Ethylene Oxide gas, and Gamma radiation shot. Hereby, we will consider Ethylene oxide sterilization.

Polypropylene pharmaceutical grade is used because of its high clarity and durability provided that recycled material is prohibited.

4.1.2 International Regulations

The International Organization for Standardization ISO published a series of documents regarding the quality, specifications and tests for plastic syringes (Table 1).

Table 4-1: ISO standards documents

International standard document	Sterile hypodermic syringe for single-use
ISO 7886-1: 2017-05	Syringes for manual use.
ISO 7886-2: 2020 E	Syringes for use with power syringes pumps.
ISO 7886-3	Auto-disabled syringes for fixed-dose immunization
ISO 7886-4: 2018-E	Syringes with re-use prevention feature

4.1.3 Components of the Syringe

Disposable syringe is considered to be of 3 units Figure 1:

1-Unit 1: barrel: a cylindrical tube with nozzle at the top serves as a needle adapter on which the hub should be fixed. Having a finger flange at the end to support the barrel during pressing of the plunger. The barrel should be of high clarity as glass with clear scale of stable ink.

Figure 4-1: Syringe components

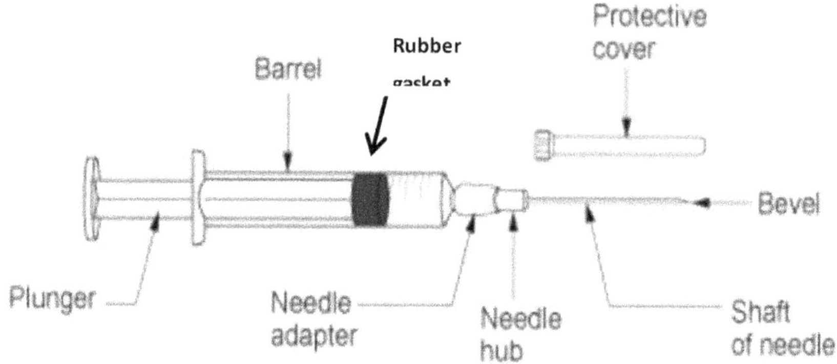

2-Unit 2:

The plunger which is stiffer and thicker, a rubber gasket is fixed at the head of the plunger. The gasket acts as a stopper preventing leakage of air or liquid and help in emptying the cylinder. At the lower part it is ended by flange on the size of the thumb. The thumb push the plunger while the two fingers hold the cylinder.

3-Unit 3:

The stainless-steel beveled needle fixed on a coloured hub by means of a suitable adhesive material and covered by a polypropylene cap to secure the needle.

Figure 4-2 shows the individual parts of the syringe.

Figure 4-2: the individual parts of the syringe.

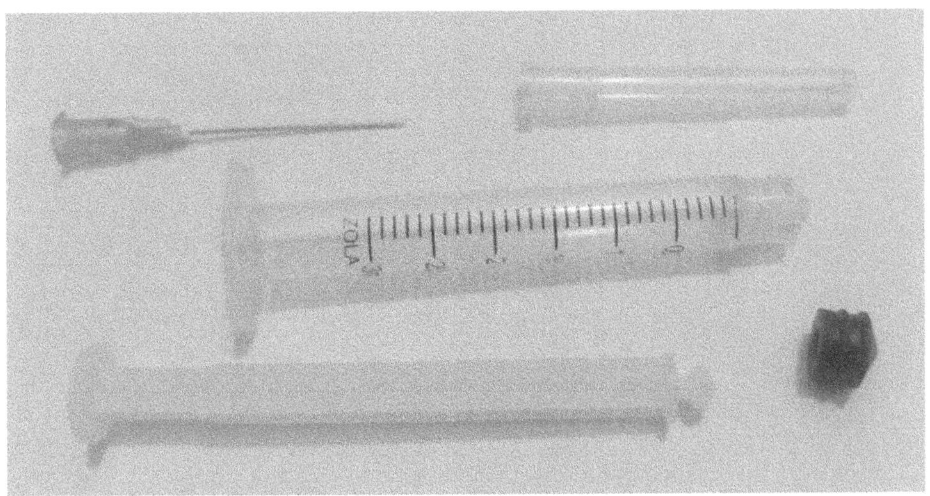

4.2 Production

All feasibility studies for the manufacturing of disposable syringes depends mainly on the production capacity of machineries, that is because of the low cost of the product. All steps of production must be relative to each other.

4.2.1 Machines and Ancillaries:

1- PP-Injection molding machines Figure 6.

2- Rubber molding machine.

3- Crushing or granulating machine, figure 7.

4- Printing machines.

5- Needle assembling line.

6- Syringe assembling machine.

7- Blister packing machine.

8- ETO sterilization Chamber.

9- Set of Moulds for the different components figure 8.

10- Loading instruments.

11- Air compressor.

12- Water or chilling source.

13- Coloured containers to collect the components.

4.2.2 Materials:

1- Polypropylene homopolymer medical grade granules, Figure 3.

2- Natural/ butyl /bromobutyl rubber. Figure 4.

3- Printing Ink.

4- Stainless steel beveled needles.

5- Adhesive material.

6- Pack paper and PVC or PP sheet.

7- Silicon oil.

8- ETO supply containers.

9- Cardboard boxes and cartons.

Figure 4-3, Polypropylene granules

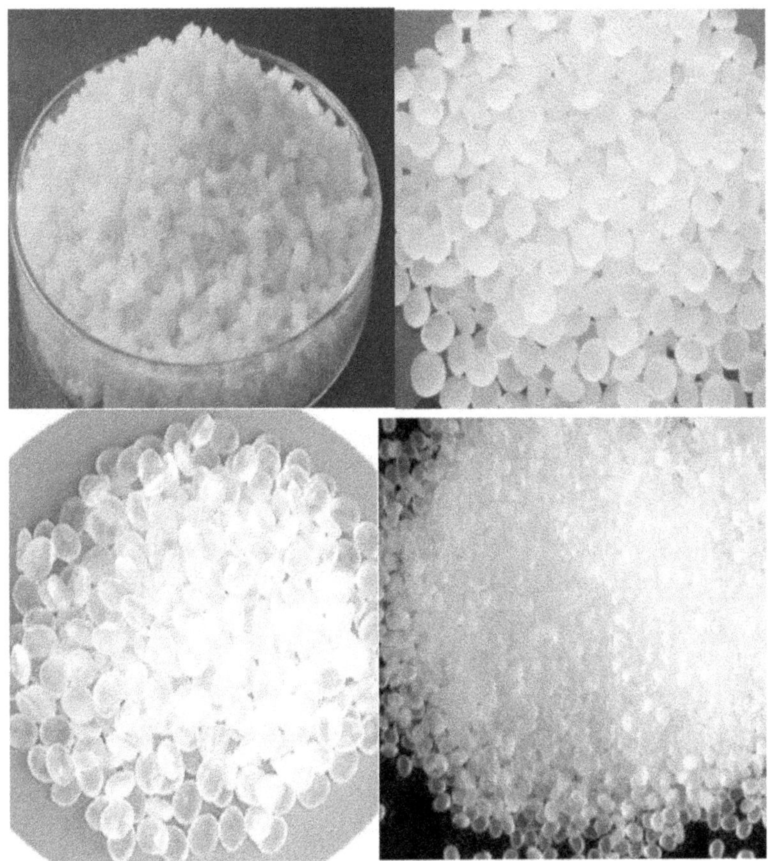

Figure 4-4 Rubber for gasket

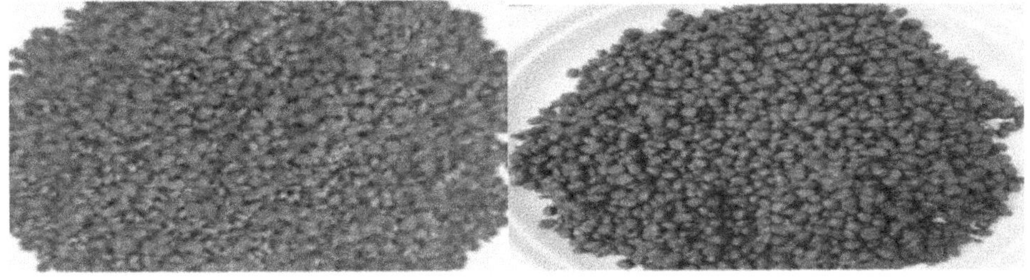

4.2.3 Production Process

Figure 4-5: Syringe manufacturing process diagram

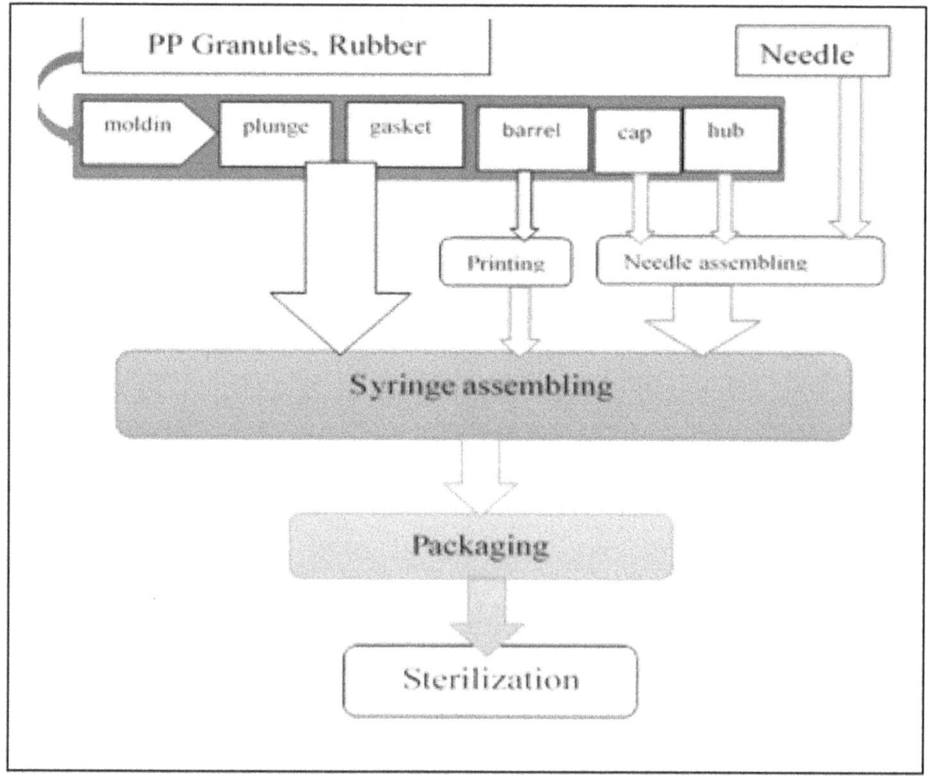

4.2.4 Injection Molding

Polypropylene is a translucent, odourless, non-toxic semi-crystalline thermoplastic, of high strength and good insulation properties. It have a low water absorbance 0.01% and density 0.89 – 0.91 of melting point 160 – 170 °C and decomposes at 350 °C having a high heat deflection temperature. It is present in copolymer and homopolymer. Homopolymer is generally used for medical purposes and it is steam sterilizable.

Polypropylene is to be fed from a hopper, dried, melted and injected to the mould then under chilling condition it will result in the shape of the mould.

For barrel design the conditions are as shown in table 4-2.

Table 4-2: Injection moulding conditions

Melting temperature	238-193 °C
Rear temperature	160-180°C
Middle temperature	180-200°C
Front temperature	200-220°C
Nozzle temperature	200-230°C
Mold temperature	60-80°C
Injection pressure	40-70 MPa
Injection time	20-60 sec.
Cooling time	20-60 sec.
Cycle time	20 sec.

→ Avoid froth, foam and bubble formation due to high speed injection. It will be avoided by low speed injection and high temperature.

→ Use a higher pressure 1500 – 1800 bar as injection pressure and 80% of it as holding pressure.

→ Temperature should not exceed 275 °C and better to be adjusted at 240°C.

→ Recycled material should not exceed 15%.

Figure 4-6: injection molding machine
[Haijian machinery manufacturing – Yinzhou, China]

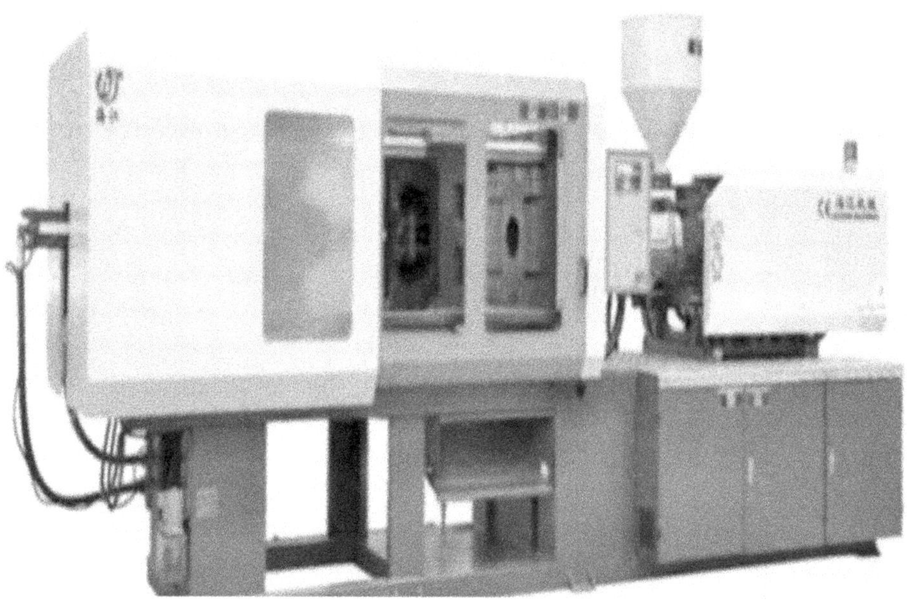

The machine should have a built-in melting system and chilling system.

For the rubber or PVC for the gasket, there should be a crushing or granulating machine as in figure 7. Gasket may be from rubber, PVC of suitable elasticity or the plunger may be without gasket especially for latex-sensitive patients.

Figure 4-7: PVC & Rubber Crushing machine
[LV HUA – Zhejiang, China]

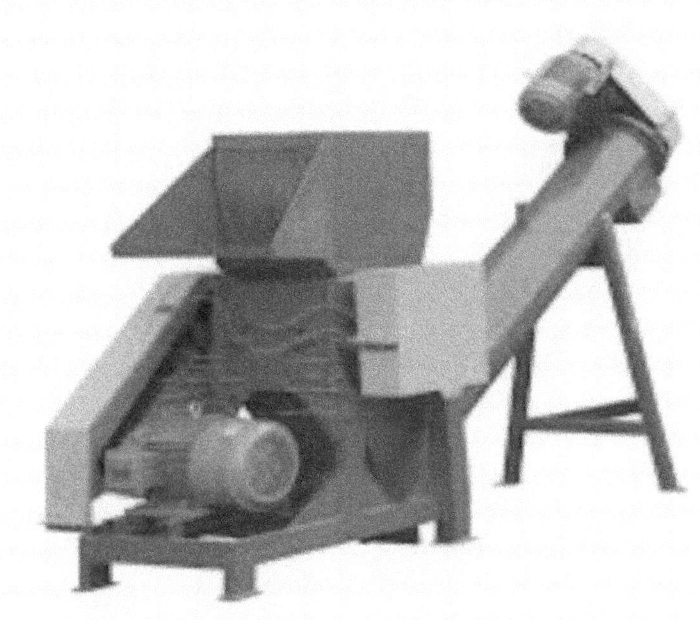

The injection molding machine can be used to produce barrels, caps, hubs, plungers and gaskets.

Molds are structured from stainless seal to produce a different number of pieces. Figure 4-8a/b/c/d shows examples of molds with the relative produced gasket.

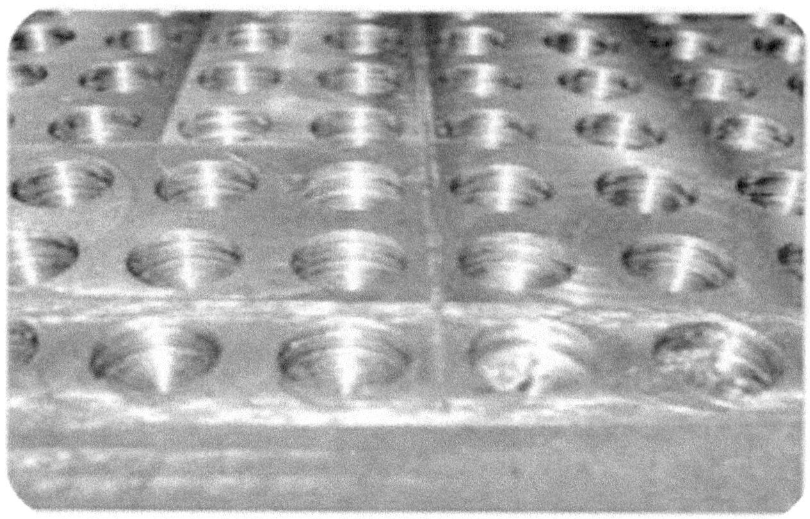

Figure 4-8a: gasket mould and its gasket product

4-8b: Stainless steel mold for production of syringe barrels

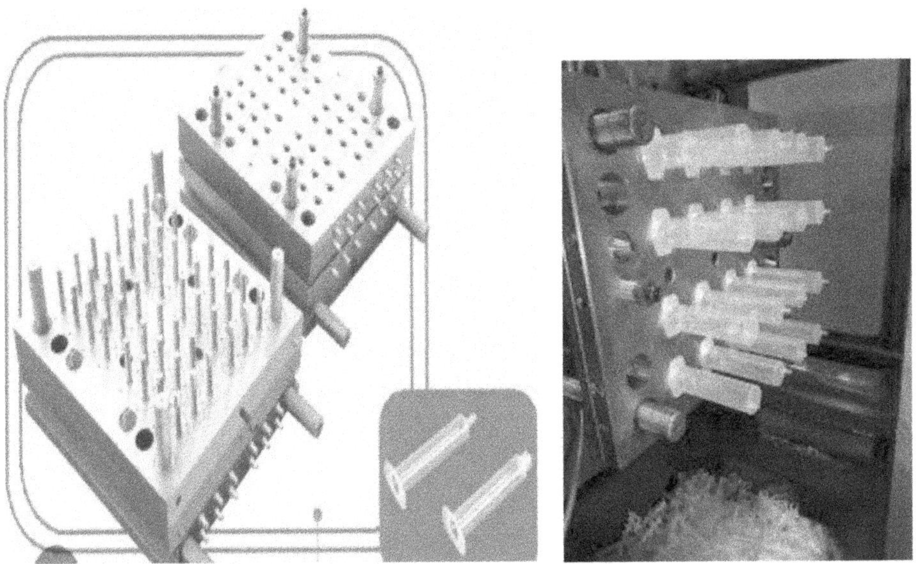

Inner side barrel mold 4-8c: Plunger Mold

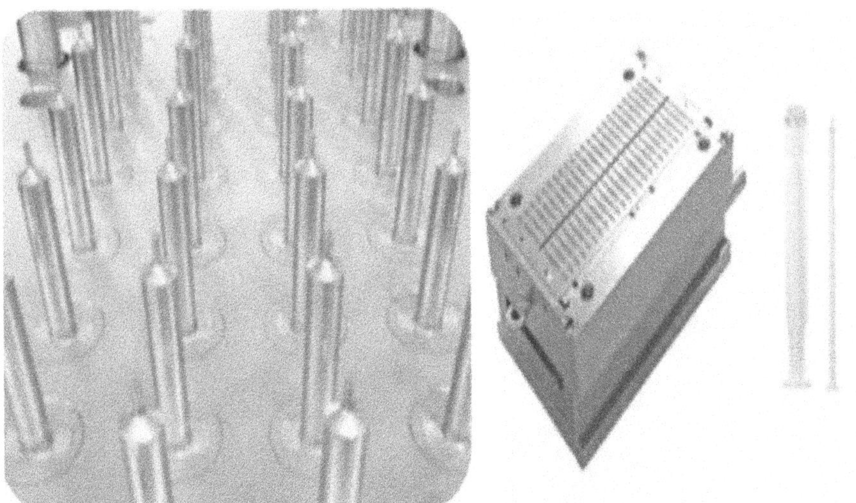

Figure 4-8d: Hub and hub mold

Hub mold hub

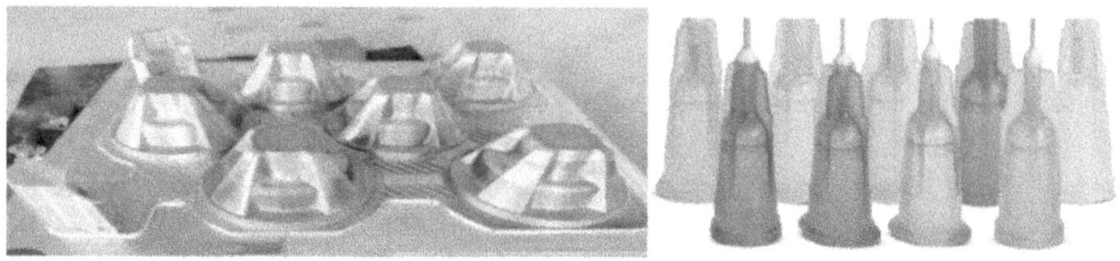

Plunger:

The plunger is the movable shaft inside the barrel which may be fitted with gasket or without. It moves outwards to suck the contents through the needle or move inwards to deliver the content through the needle. The position of the plunger inside the barrel represents the volume of the content and a measure of the dose control. It somewhat more hard and tough than the barrel. It ends with the thumb rest where the user places his thumb to press in the plunger.

4.2.5 Printing of Barrel

The second step for the barrel is to scale it into ml or units as in the case of insulin syringes. The graduation took place in a printer machine using special ink. The printing machine should be accurate and 360° printing range and precise at all times.

The ink used should have the following specifications:

1/ Not toxic, free from heavy metals.

2/ Precise, sharp, visible with no errors.

3/ must be able to dry fast enough just to transfer to the barrel surface.

4/ Must be opaque, fast adhesive and dry quickly.

5/ must comply all medical regulations.

If the ink shows slower dryness, it will get smudged and if it is too fast it will dry on the steel roller or the rubber roller. To print properly, the surface tension of the substrate must be greater than the surface tension of the ink. So, the barrel may undergo corona treatment

There are many types of barrel printers of which are:

1/ rotary syringe or rotary pad printer (figure 4-9).

2/ automatic screen printer (figure 4-10).

Ink is applied on an engraved roller. The rubber roller or the screen came into contact with the moving barrel where the engraved ink is stamped or the screen is copied.

Figure 4-9: Rotary Syringe printer *[Spinks-Indianmart.com]*

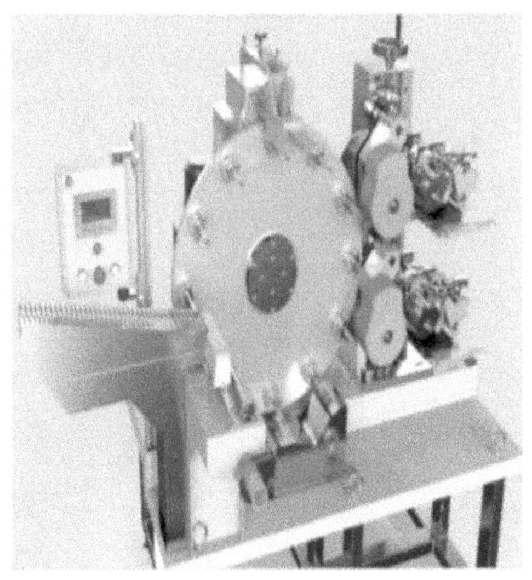 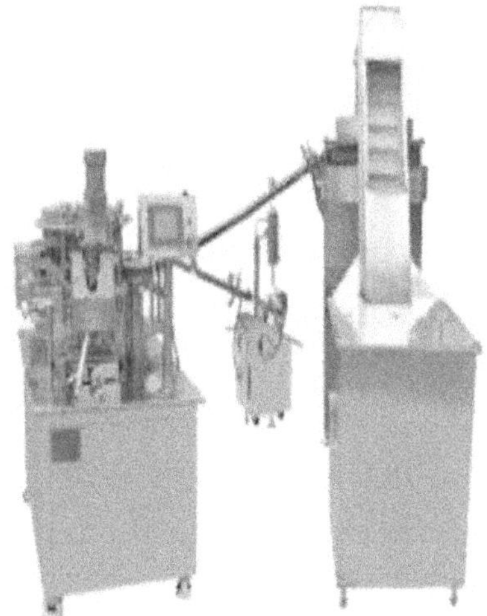

Figure 4-10: Automatic screen printer

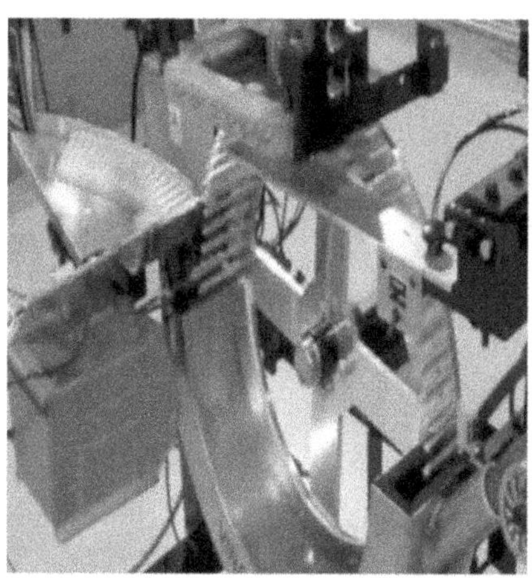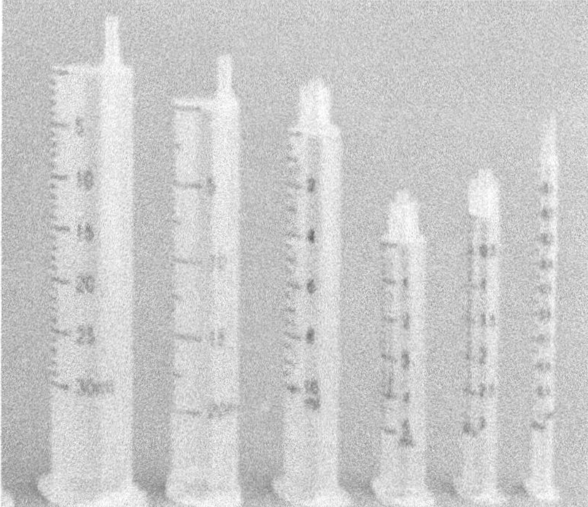

The barrel should be transparent to allow viewing of the fluid inside and match it to the printed scale. For this reason, fresh medical grade PP should be used without any recycled portion.

The graduation interval generally 0.2 ml – 0.5 ml and the graduation line is 1 ml volume. The barrel should be of volume 10% more than the nominal capacity.

The nozzle may be centric or eccentric that is to say it may be situated in the center or peripherally situated. The luer slip also may be central or eccentric. The eccentric is better for the intravenous or intra-arterial injection.

The luer-lock may be screw lock or twisting lock which can prevent the movement of the needle from the barrel making a secure use of syringe.

4.2.6 Corona Treatment

Corona discharge is an electrical discharge caused by the ionization of air surrounding by a conductor carrying a high voltage. The corona discharge occurs at locations where the strength of the electrical field exceeds the dielectric strength of air. This treatment leads to increase in the surface tension rendering the surface suitable for adhesion of ink in the case of barrel printing or adhesion of an adhesive material as in case of needle-hub bonding.

Figure 4-11: corona treater [PRM-Taiwan]

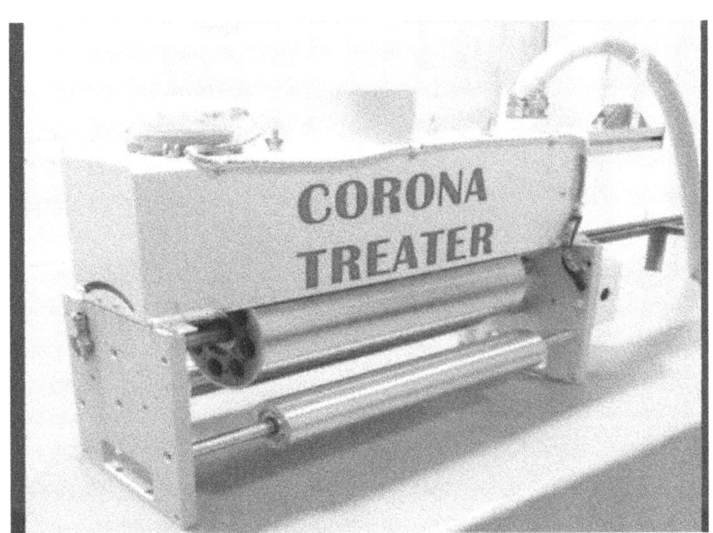

The gasket

May be made of rubber, PVC or silicon. It is fitted to the plunger head. Inside the barrel, it protects from leakage of fluid or air to the inside and outside the barrel and provides a smooth movement of the plunger.

4.3 The Needle

4.3.1 Needle Manufacture

The needle generally produced at specific factory and not at the syringe factory. Although all quality control tests are performed at the manufacturer laboratories but results should be confirmed at the syringe manufacturing facility.

hypodermic needles

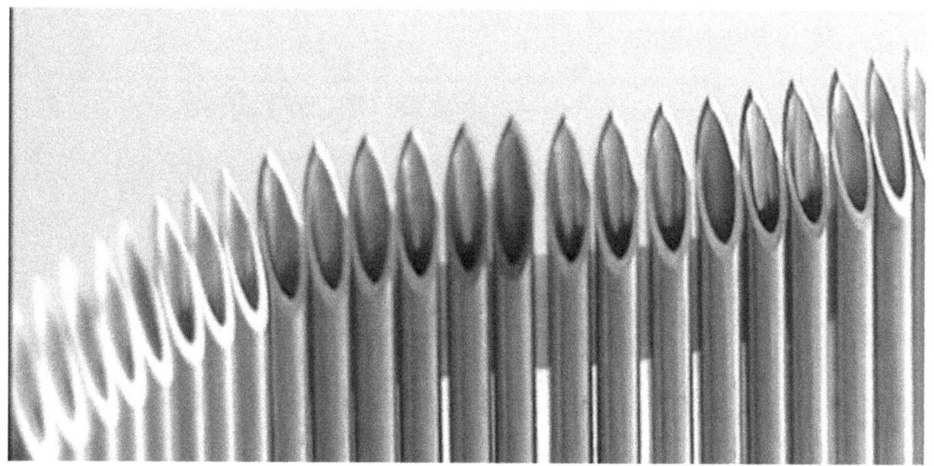

The hypodermic needles usually manufactured at specialized factory. There are usually packed in 500,000 needles in a small box. The needle consists of a hollow needle tube and different lengths with beveled sharp point. Usually, of smooth surfaces lubricated by silicon oil.

Figure 4-12: Manufacturing process diagram of needles.

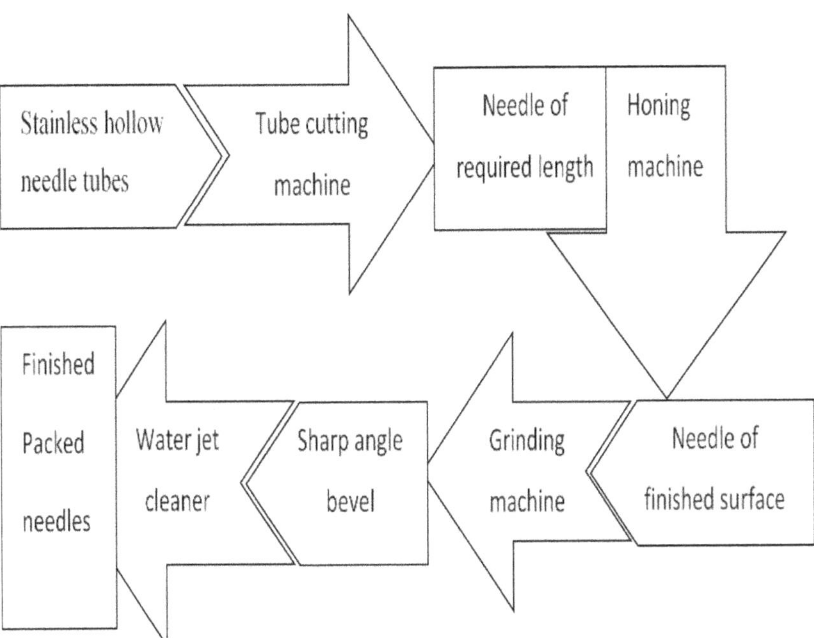

4.3.2 Needle Gauge and Length

The gauge is an international standard to express the diameter of the needle lumen. However, the smaller the gauge the larger the lumen and as the gauge increases, the needle is thinner.

Table 3-4 shows the international gauges, the length of the needle and the appropriate use with the relevant hub color.

(P.T.O)

Table 4-3 The gauge, the length in inches and uses of needle.

Gauge	Length	Uses	Hub color
16	1.5	Infusion surgery & trauma	White
18	1.5	Critical care	Pink
19	1.5	Critical care	Cream
20	1.5	Drawing from vial I.V	Yellow
21	1.5	I.V	Green
22	1.5	I.M for children, adult and geriatric.	Black
23	1.5	I.M for children and adult	Blue
24	1.5	I.M for children and adult.	Medium purple
22	1	I.M for infants and children.	
23	1	I.M for infant and children.	
24	1	I.M for infants and neonates.	
25	1	I.M for infants and neonates.	Orange
26	0.5	Ophthalmic and intradermal.	Brown
27	0.5	Ophthalmic and intradermal.	Medium grey
26	1.5	Dental.	
27	0.5	Dental.	

4.3.3 The Hub

The hub is the base of the needle where it it is bonded by an appropriate adhesive material. It is often coloured according to the standard color code which indicates the gauge of the needle. The pantone ISO 6009 color standard is used. The hub is either slipped fit to the luer or screw or twisting fit to the nozzle of the cylinder.

The hub is generally corona treated during the process of needle assembling to facilitate the bonding of the adhesive material between the hub and the base of the needle.

4.3.4 The Needle Cap

The needle cap is produced by injection molding machine and fitted to the needle at the last step of the assembling. It provides a protective cover for the needle and protection of personnel handling the needle.

4.3.5 Needle Assembling Process

At this step, 3 components are to be assembled on one-line machine. The needle, the hub and the needle cap. This requires a series of highly sophisticated technicalities

Needle assembling process requires the assembling of three parts to produce one syringe components. The three parts are the needle to be connected with the hub and covered by the cap. It is a very sophisticated electronic process with electronic sensors for the inspection and direction of the needle and the hub and application of the adhesive glue (figures 4-13& 4-14). It is essential to safeguard the process, the needle and the operators.

Figure 4-13: Automatic needle assembling line
[BS Medical Co Ltd-S. Korea]

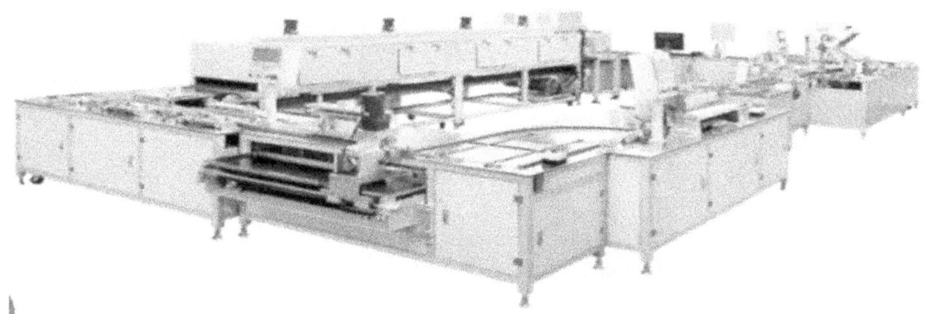

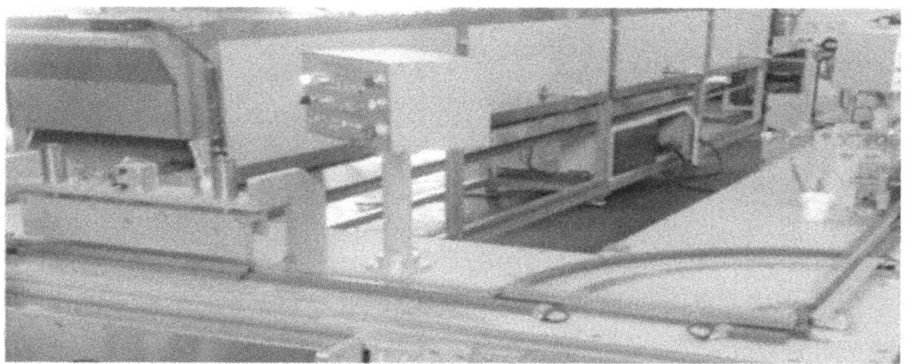

Figure 4-14: Needle assembling process diagram

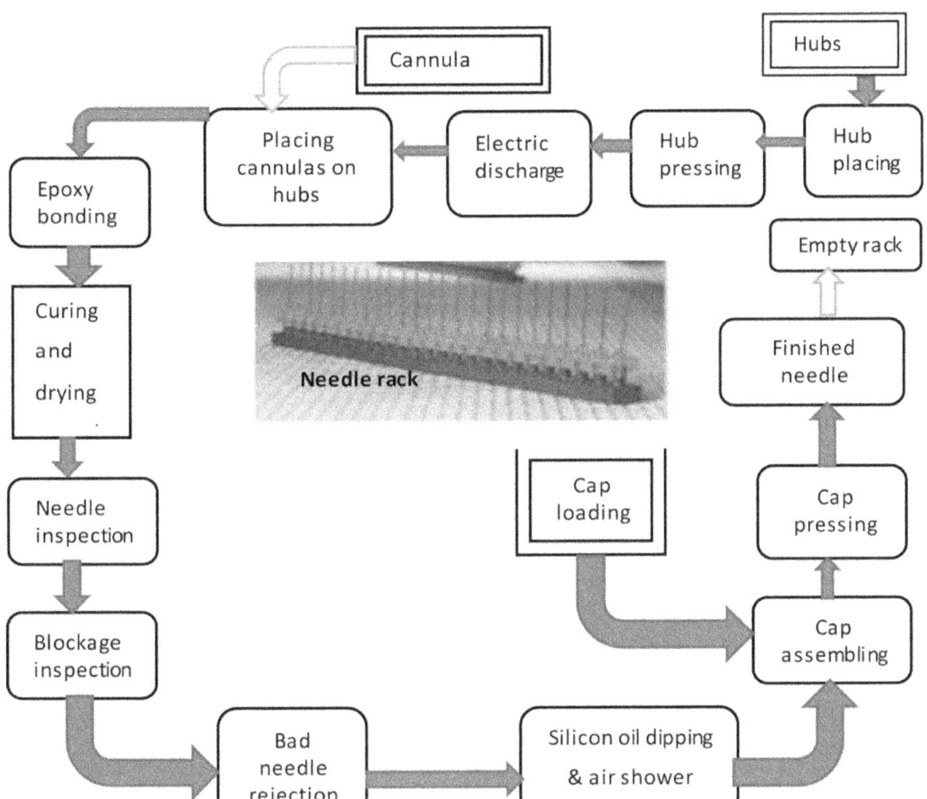

Remarks on the process

→ Because PP surface is very smooth and the surface of the hub is shiny and glazy, it requires corona treatment at-line. Therefore, the needle hub requires an electric discharge (high voltage sparking) before the application of the glue to secure the adhesion of the needle cannula to the hub.

→ Siliconization process take place by raising a container containing medical grade silicon oil upwards while inverting the rack holding the needles downwards allowing dipping. Then followed by air shower to remove any droplet of the oil and uniformly distribute the oil on the needle surface. This siliconization facilitate the penetration of the needle and its movement inside the body tissue.

→ The adhesive epoxy resin is a polymer compounds such as master bond adhesives/ sealants. It should prevent fluid leakage, secure a fixed position of the cannula to the hub and it should be fast cure as one part; no fragmentation with excellent depth cure and easily automated. It should be solvent free composite of enough hardness and toughness. The ISO 7884: 2016 defines the specifications for the bond strength between the hub and the cannula as MED-NPT-200N.

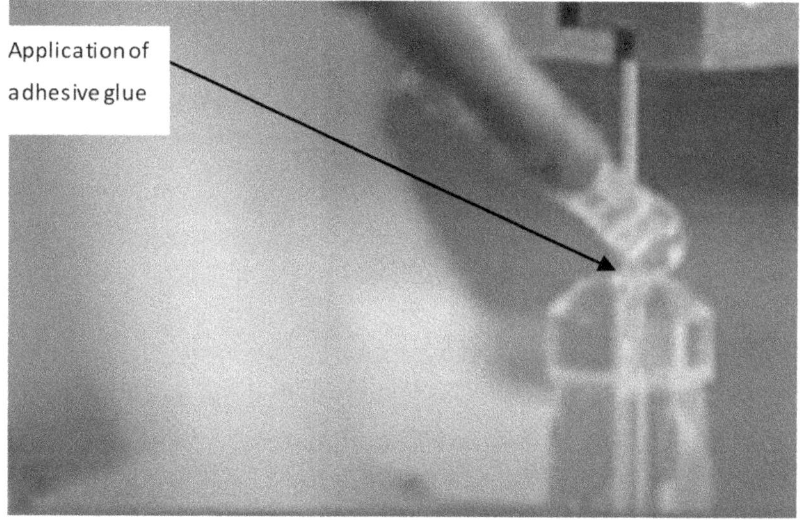

At-line inspection:

Inspection during assembling may be optical, digital or measurement. Some lines use Lynx EVO with 360° viewer and camera as optical inspection system. Others use DRV-ZI 3D digital viewer with 200 zoom and ability to share images or videos in real time to off-site location or local display. Measurement TVM – rapid video field of view system. There are some dual optical and digital video inspection and measurement system.

Bad needle may be rejected using Keyence CCD image system having speed of 45 pieces per second for detection of unqualified needles.

4.4 Syringe Assembling Process

This process involves the assembling of the printed syringe barrel, the finished needle, the gasket and the plunger.

The automatic line is composed from three parts, one part assembling the barrel to the finished needle. The second parts inserting the plunger head into the gasket cavity and the third part concerned with the insertion of the headed plunger into the barrel holding the needle. Some of the automatic lines can be fed automatically from the printing machine and other are fed manually. In some lines the lubricating silicon oil is sprayed into the barrel or dropped during the printing process and some lines adopts spraying or dropping of oil during the assembling process. Syringe assembling involves the following steps figure 4-15A, 4-15B, 4-15C and 4-15D:

1- Inserting the plunger into the gasket cavity by pressing.

2- Fixing needle with the barrel and silicon oil spraying.

3- Plunger with gasket is inserted into the barrel with the needle.

4- Ejected as assembled syringe ready for packaging.

Figure 4-15A Automatic syringe assembling line
[SMARTEL-China]

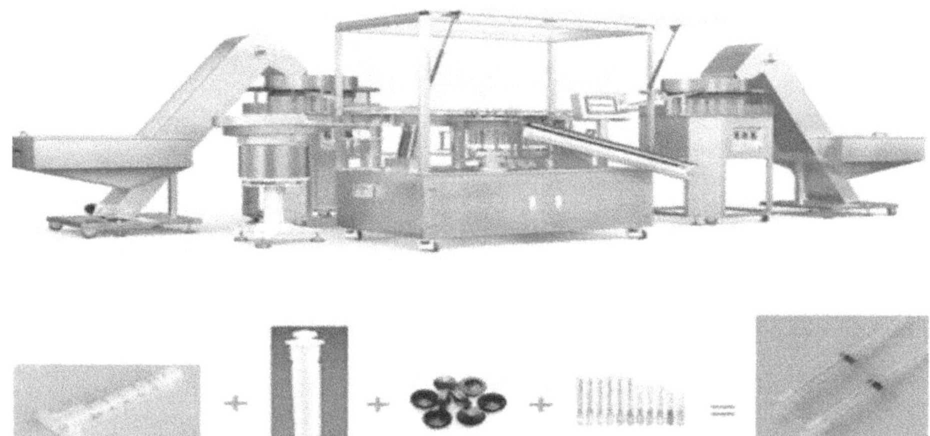

Figure 4-15 B: Syringe assembling machine
[Yuhuan Hengxiang Machinery Equipment, syringeassemblymachine.com]

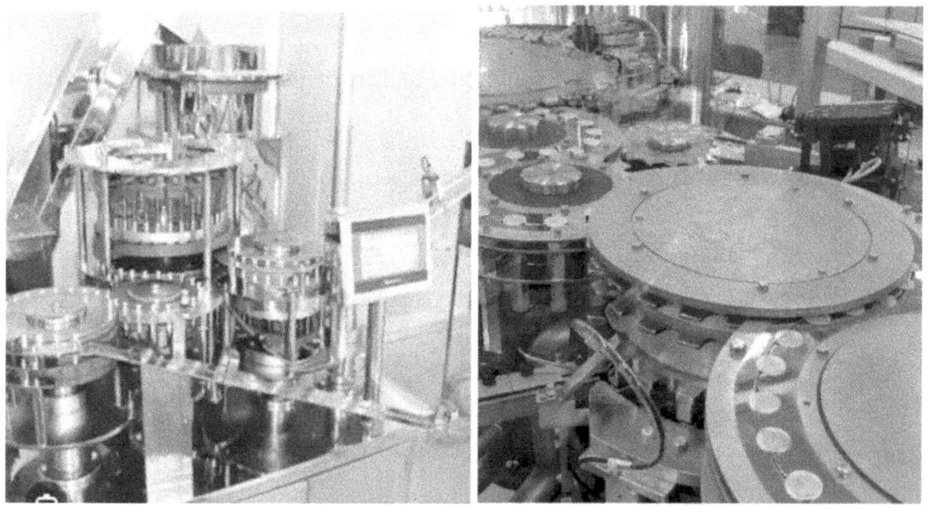

Figure 4-15 C: Last step in assembling machine
[Taizhou Maidike Int-China & Kahle automation-Italy]

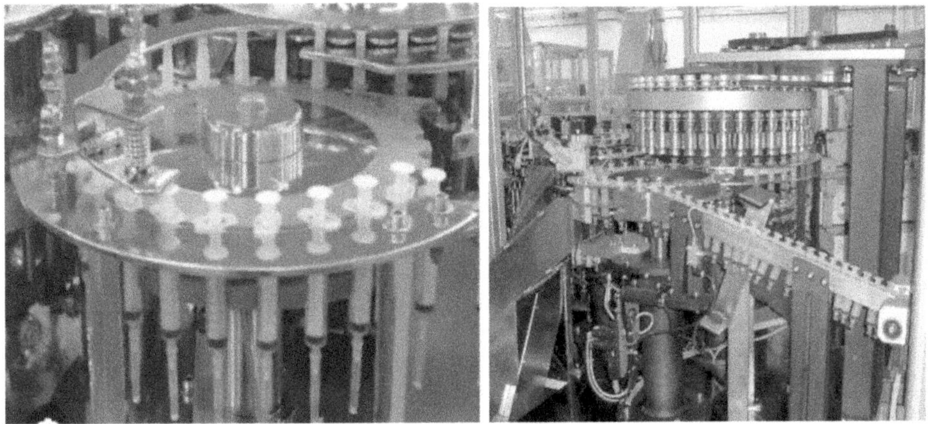

Figure 4-15 D: syringe assembling parts

Step 1: four parts

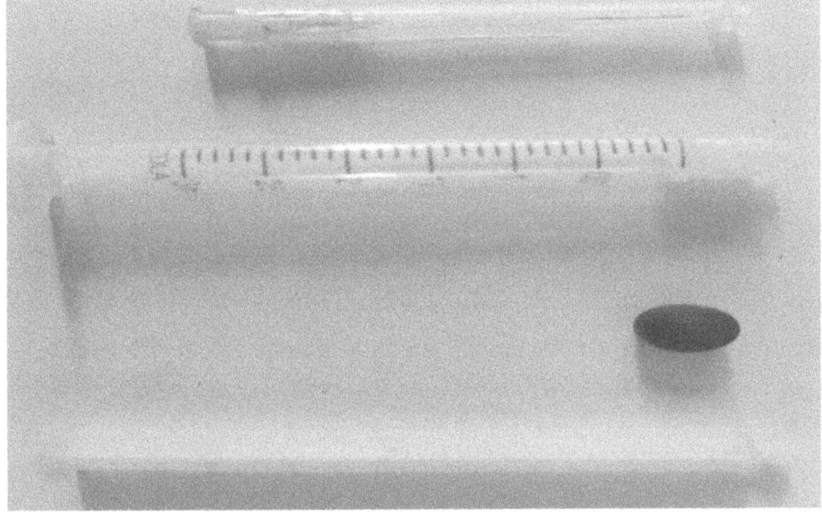

Step 2: two parts

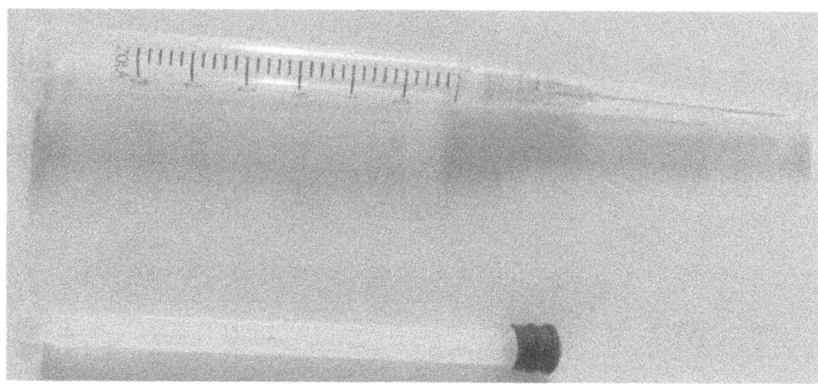

Final step: one single syringe

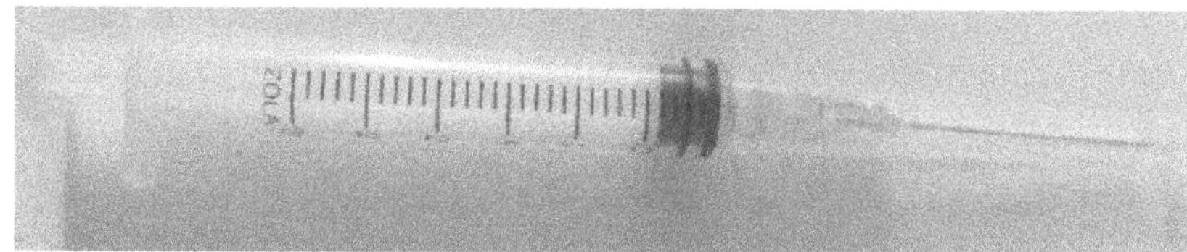

4.5 Packaging of Syringe

Syringe packaging is in paper/ plastic composite. Paper is already printed and treated to accept heat sealing. The machine is provided with cavities (figure 4-16a), a printer to print the lot number, the manufacture and expiration dates.

Syringes are either fed automatically or manually by hand (figure 4-16b). The plastic sealable membrane is placed over the mould and a heat suction by vacuum is applied and then syringes are placed into the deep drawing cavities of the convoying mould (figure 4-16c).

There may be a syringe lifter to place the syringes into the cavities. Upper heating system may be applied to make the film more uniform and elegant. The heat seal mechanism involves heating system, heat seal air-bag, heat seal mould, lifting and screw displacement.

After sealing the paper to the plastic membrane, the colour sealer sensor defines the transverse cutting with rolling cutting mode (figure 4-16d. T

Then then the cut syringes are packed (figure 4-16e).

Figure 4-16a: Packing machine with cavities *[Smartell]*

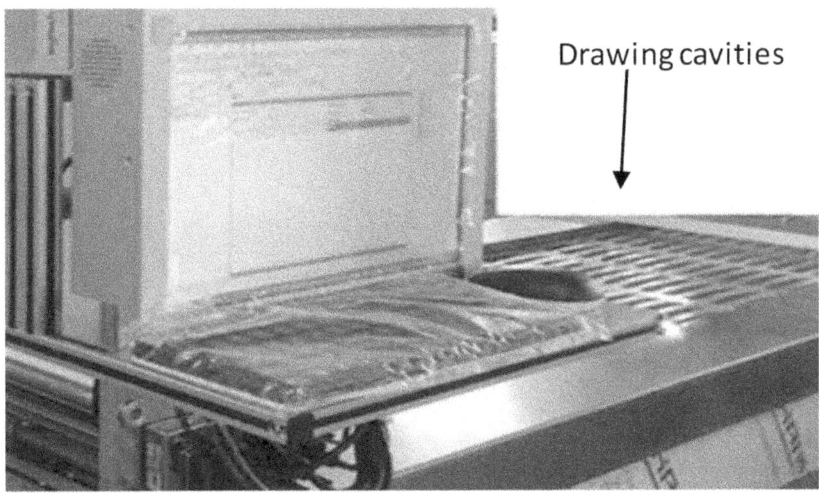

Figure 4-16-b: placing syringes by hand

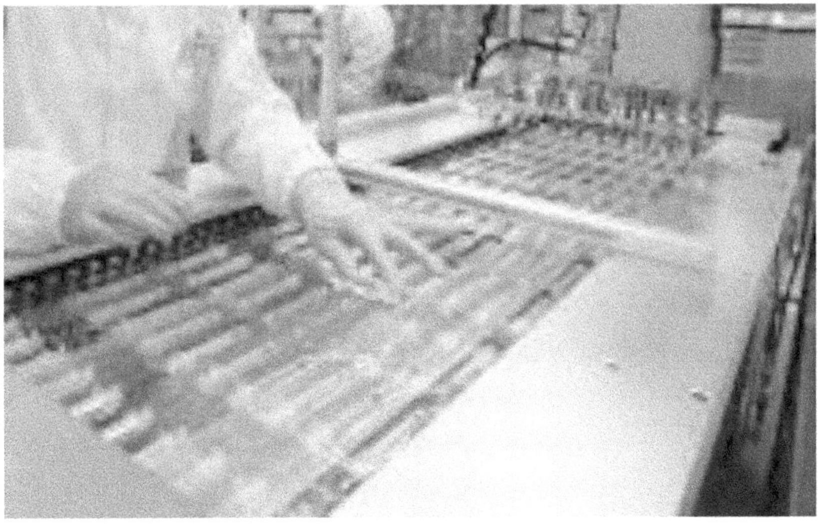

Figure 4-16-c Arranging the paper pack

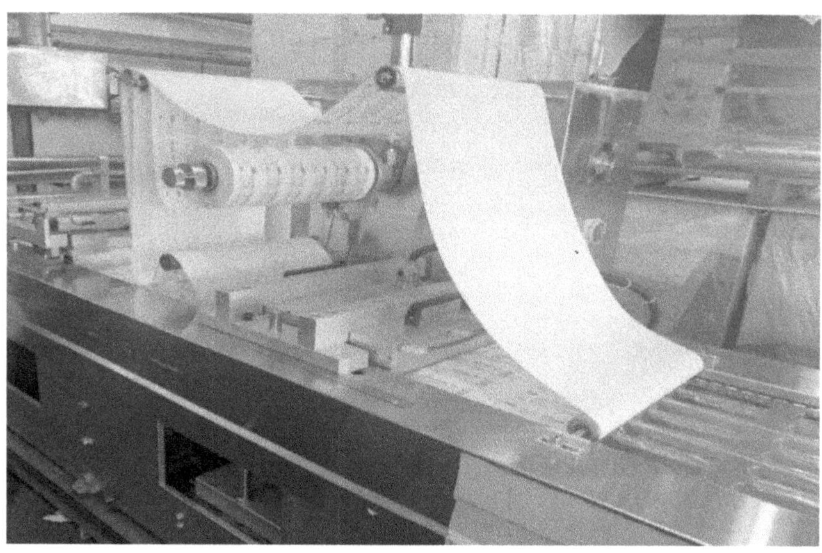

Figure 4-16-d: Roller cutting

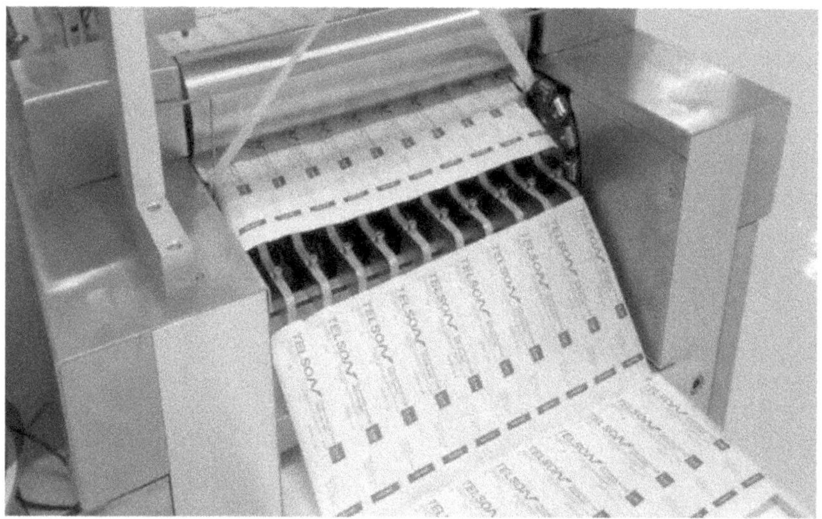

Figure 4-16e: Packed syringes

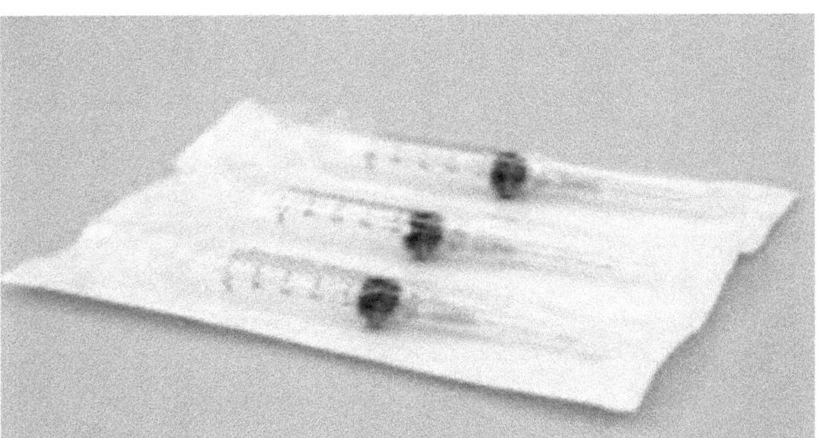

Then the packed syringes are placed into card board boxes in 100s, fifties or 25s according to the required box quantity.

4.6 Sterilization

Generally, sterilization is carried out by gamma radiation shot or ethylene oxide gas. Sterilization by ethylene oxide gas is carried out at the level of the factory scale in a suitable size champers (figure 4-17).

Ethylene oxide has a high penetration power causing alkalization of the bacterial essential metabolite of the reproductive system leading to its death.

4.6.1 Factors Governing Sterilization by Ethylene Oxide Gas

There are four factors governing the sterilization process by ethylene oxide:

1- The concentration of the gas which should be 450-1200 mg/litre volume.

2- The temperature which should be 37–63 °C.

3- The humidity which should be 40–80% RH.

4- The process duration which should be 1-6 hours.

In practice, 65% humidity and 55°C and vacuum of 27 inch of Hg for 3 hours may be sufficient to kill the existing bacteria.

After sterilization, the products require aeration for 8–12 hours at least at 50-60°C. So, the steps of ethylene oxide are as follows:

1- Preconditioning and humidification up to 98% for one hour or longer.

2- Gas introduction.

3- Exposure.

4- Evacuation of chamber.

5- Air washes for 2.5 hours.

6- Aeration for 8-12 hours.

Figure 4-17 – (A,B,C) Gas sterilization chamber

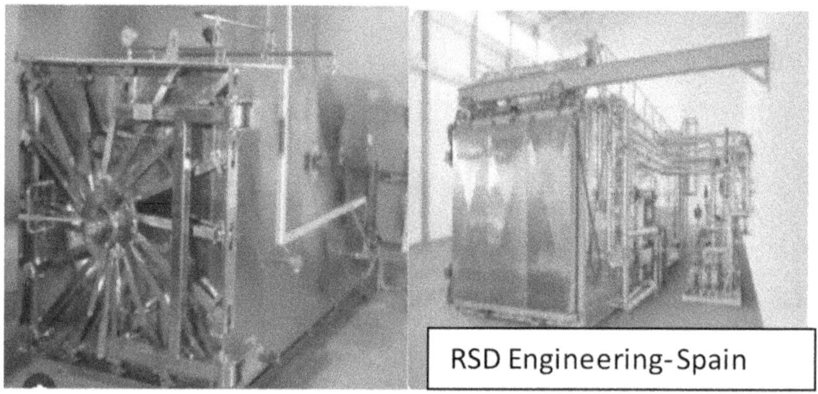

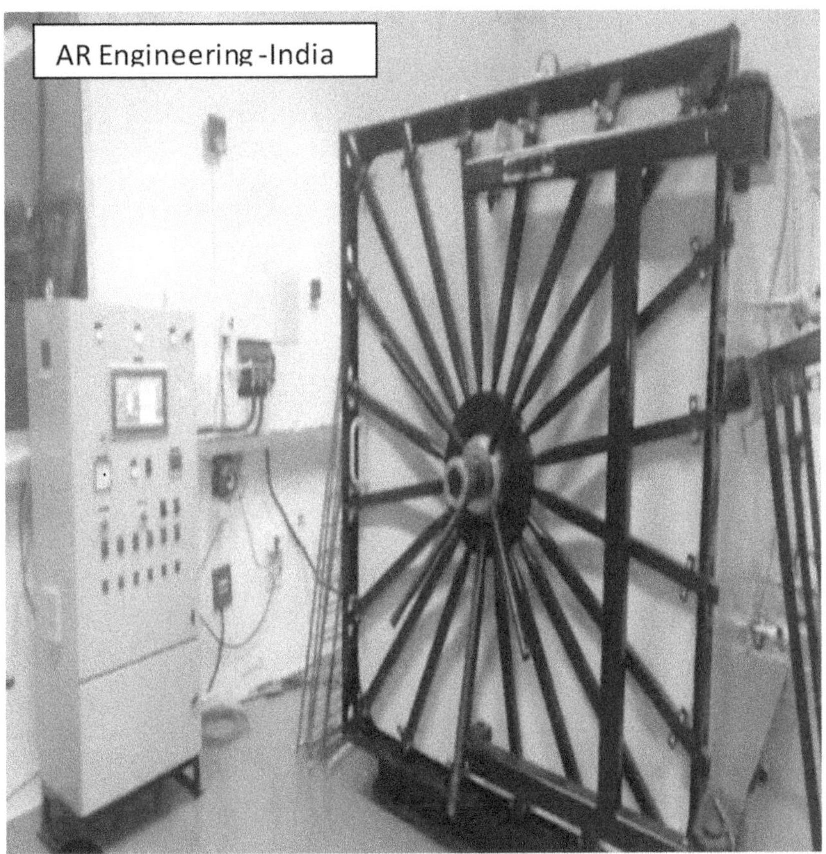

Ethylene oxide is an inflammable and explosive gas. It is heat sensitive, so, it should be handles with caution. It is supplied in cylinders and transported under controlled and regulated conditions. Figure 18 shows some ETO cylinders. Data sheet should be accompanied during shipment.

Figure 4-18: Ethylene oxide gas Cylinders – dryice.co.in,
Indianmart. Qingdao Ludong Gas-china]

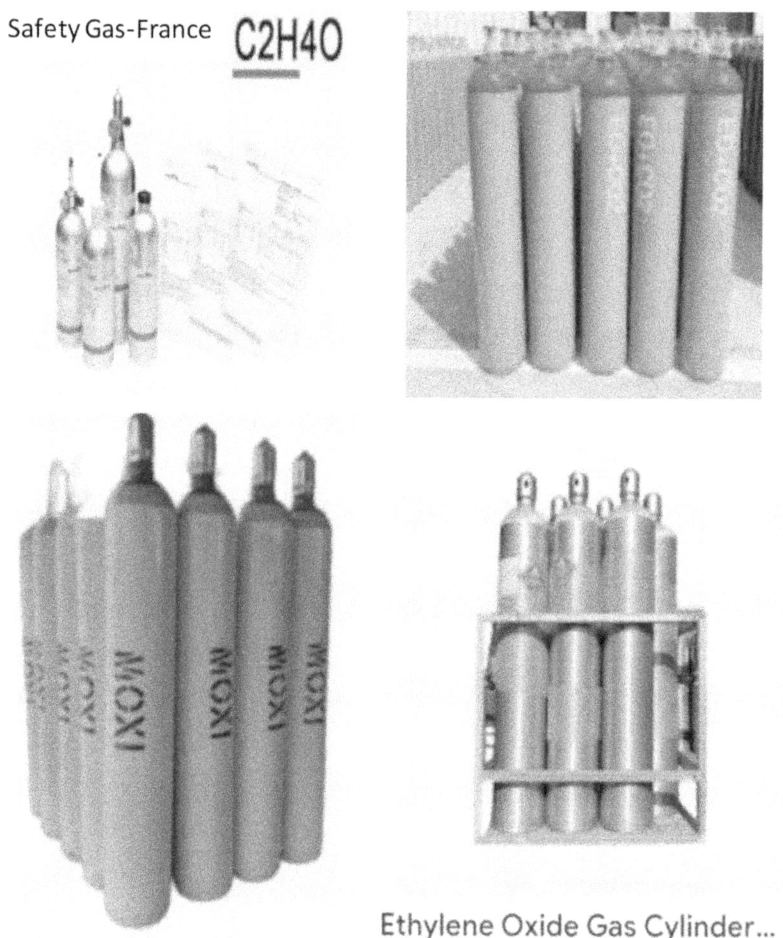

4.6.2 Indicators for Ethylene Oxide Sterilization

4.6.2.1 Chemical indicators

There are many types and brands of chemical indicators for ETO sterilization process. All indicators are based on change of colour when exposed to ETO sterilization conditions.

- Class 1 indicators change colours when exposed to sterilization process.

- Class 2 indicators change colour depending on the sterilization conditions providing more detailed information based on the sterilization parameters.

- Also, some indicators change colour based on combination of temperature and time and ETO concentration (figure 4-19).

Chemical indicators contain dyes that change colour at a certain range of temperature, when it is subjected to ETO sterilization, it reacts with the sterilization conditions and undergo visible changes indicating that the sterilization process is successful. This requires that the indicator should be perfectly placed into the chamber.

(P.T.O)

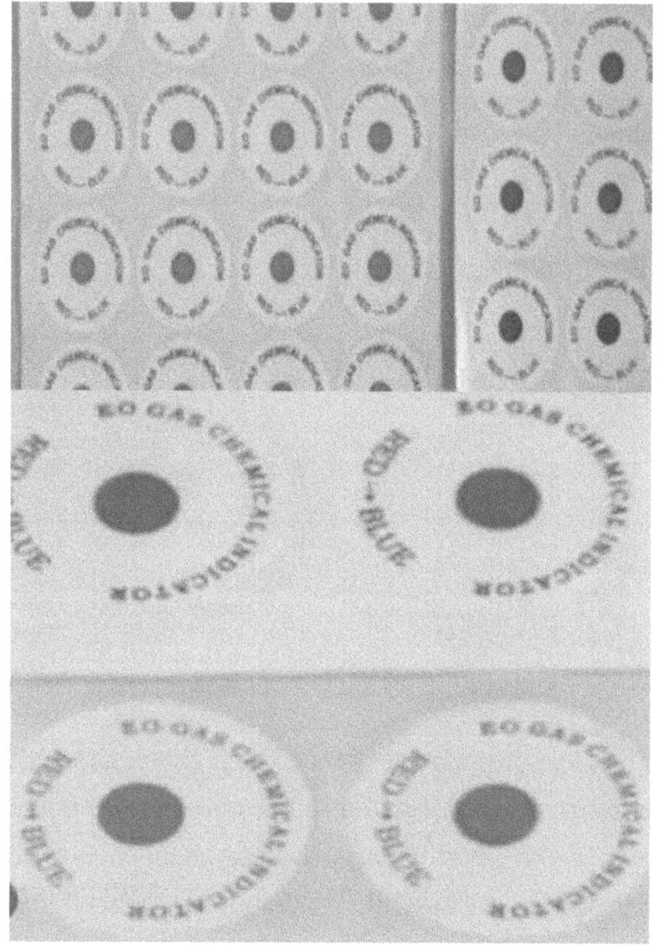

Figure 4-19: Chemical Indicators – *Roshan Rai Sepahan*

4.6.2.2 Biological indicators

Biological indicators for ETO sterilization process consist of a *Bacillus atrophaeus* spore strip with growth medium and bromothymol blue as pH indicator dye system. The biological indicator is activated after the sterilization process and join the growth media with the process spore strip. The biological indicator incubated for 48 hours (depending on the instructions). Changing of colour from green to yellow indicates bacterial growth, that means the test is positive and the sterilization is inefficient.

In some indicators the indicators is a special filter paper inoculated with *bacillus atrophaeus*. The biological indicators is used to validate or qualify the sterilization process according to USP standard specifications and ISO 11138-2. The incubation temperature is 30-35°C for 7 days. Change in colour from red to yellow or turbidity indicates microbial growth. Figure 4-20 demonstrate two brand of biological indicators and change in color.

The incubation period and the resultant change in colour depends on the manufacturer instructions and the indicators may be discs or strips. But usually not re-usable.

Figure 4-20: biological indicators and change in colour

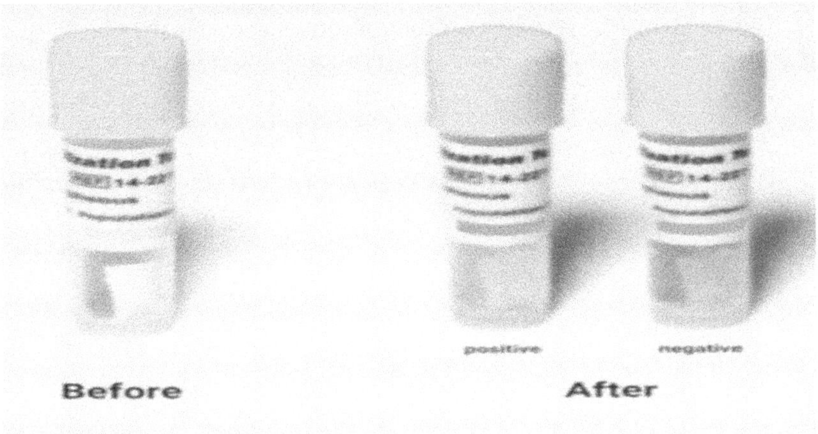

After finishing the sterilization cycle, the chamber is washed to get rid of ethylene oxide and the dissolve it in water and discharged.

Then the sterilized product is placed for aeration for the longest possible time at least 8 – 12 hours to eliminate the residual ethylene oxide as shown in figure 4-021.

Figure 4-21: Products in the chamber and aeration

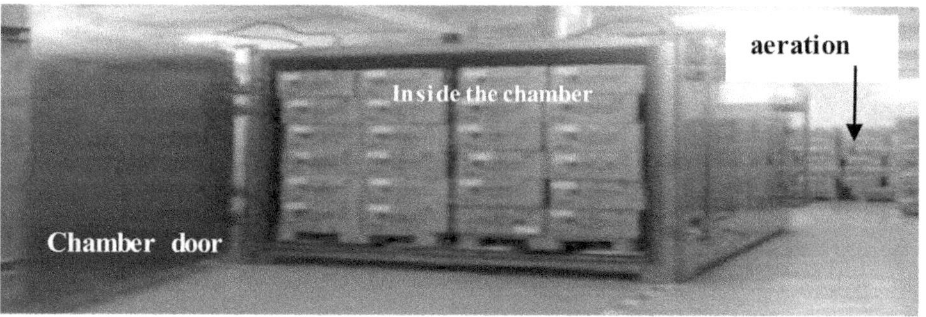

Section 5:

Requirements and Tests for Single Use Syringes

5. Regulatory Overview

The *Ph.Eur* defines the sterile single-use plastic syringes as medical devices intended for immediate use for administration of injectable preparations. They are supplied sterile and pyrogen-free and are not to be re-sterilised or re-used. They consist of a syringe barrel and a piston which may have elastomer sealing ring; they may be fitted with a needle which may be not detachable. Each syringe is presented with individual protection for maintaining sterility. According to this definition, there are two main parts, the syringe and the needle. The International Organization for Standardization ISO presents documents ISO 7864 for the requirements and testing for the needle and ISO 7886 for the syringe body.

The tests required are physical tests regarding the barrel, plunger and stopper, the different measurement and physical parameters of both of the syringe and the needle.

Chemically, there are tests for the residual silicon oil and ethylene oxide gas remaining after sterilization. At the same time the microbiological tests regarding the sterility and the pyrogenicity remain the most essential teste for both the syringe and the needle.

5.1 Requirements and Tests for the Syringe

5.1.1 Secondary Packaging, Storage Containers and Wrapping

The following information should be printed and checked:

1- Description of the content, the nominal capacity, the type of nozzle and the quantity of syringes in the package.

2- The word " Sterile".

3- The word " For Single-Use Only".

4- Warning to check the integrity of the of the primary container before use.

5- Batch or lot number.

6- The sterilization date and the method of sterilization.

7- The name and address of the manufacturer.

8- Information for handling, storage and transportation.

5.1.2 Primary Container

1- Should be well sealed.

2- Should ensure the maintenance of sterility and cleanliness.

3- Should provide minimum risk of contamination during the opening process.

4- Should protect the syringe during normal handling.

5- Should not be re-sealed when ruptured or opened.

5.1.3 Labelling

1- Description of the content, capacity and type of nozzle.

2- The word "Sterile".

3- The word " For Single-Use Only", may use the sympol as in figure (3-1).

4-   Warning in case of incompatibility for example " Not to be used with paraldehyde".

5-   Batch number.

6-   Sterilization date and expiration date.

7-   Trade name and name and logo of the manufacturer.

Figure (5-1) ISO Symbol for not reuse

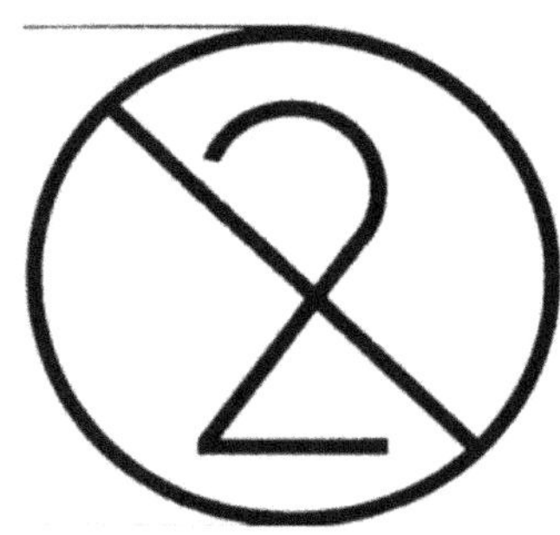

5.1.4 Graduated Scale

The syringe should have one or more scales expressing the limit of volume contained in the barrel. The scale can be extended after the nominal capacity but this extension should be distinguished from the original scale graduation.

Differentiation can be by:

a.   Circulation.

b.   Dotted line or broken line.

c.   Different colour or font size.

d.   Shorter graduation lines.

→ Lines should be symmetrical in thickness and vertical layout forming right angles with the axis of the barrel.→ The length of the shorter lines should be approximately half the length of the long lines.

→ Table 5-1 shows the tolerance on the graduated capacity, the minimum length of the scale to the nominal capacity, the interval and the increments between graduation lines to be numbered.

→ The zero-graduation line of the scale should coincide with the fiducial line on the piston within a quarter of the smallest scale interval.

→ The numbers should be close to the graduation line but not touching the line.

Table (5-1) Syringe graduation requirements

Nominal capacity V	Tolerance of capacity		Max. length scale	Scale interval	Increment between numbered lines
	Less than half V	Half or more than V			
V < 2 ml	±1.5% of v +2% of expelled volume	±5% of expelled volume	57 mm	0.05 ml	0.1 ml
2-v < 5	,,	,,	27 mm	0.2 ml	0.5 or 1
5-v < 10	±1.5% of v +1% of expelled volume	±4% of expelled volume	36	0.5	1
10-v<20	,,	,,	44	1	5
20-v<30	,,	,,	52	2	10
30-v<50	,,	,,	67	2	10
50 < V	,,	,,	75	5	10

5.1.5 The Barrel

5.1.5.1 Dimensions

The length of the barrel shall allow maximum usable capacity 10% more the nominal capacity.

5.1.5.2 Finger grips

They are flange at the open end of the barrel which should be free from sharp endings and when the syringe is placed on a horizontal surface it makes 10° and not more than 180°. The function of these flange is to enable the syringe to be held securely during its use.

5.1.5.3 The interior surface

A-Cleanliness: On visual inspection without magnification at 300-700 lx, the inner surface of the barrel should be free from particles and any extraneous matter.

B-Lubricant

On visual inspection, the lubricant should not be visible as particles or droplets. The Eur.Ph accepted undiluted polydimethylsiloxane for 3 parts syringes and the quantity should not be more than 0.25 mg/ cm^2 of the internal surface area of the syringe barrel.

For 2 parts syringes (without elastomer stopper) the accepted lubricant is fatty acid amide of ercucic and/or oleic acid and the quantity should NMT 0.6% m/m of the mass of the barrel.

<u>C-Extractable metal and pH.</u>

<u>Preparation of the test extract</u>

Fill 3 syringes to the nominal capacity with distilled water then expel the air bubbles and maintain at 37 + 0-3 °C for 8 hours + 0-15 minutes. Combine the content in borosilicate glass container. Use the remaining portion of the distilled water as a control fluid.

D-pH:

Using an electrode pH meter, the test extract should be within one unit of that of the control fluid.

Total extractable metal:

Using atomic absorption, NMT 5 mg/litre of lead, zinc and iron. Cadmium should be NMT 0.1 mg/litre.

5.1.5.4 The nozzle

The ISO 594 – 1 and ISO 594-2 specify the standards of conical and locking fitting for the nozzle. The nozzle should be centrally coaxial with the barrel for syringes of nominal capacity less than 5 ml and may be centric or eccentric for 5ml or more.

The axis of the eccentric nozzle should be of a distance from the nearest point in the internal surface of the barrel not greater than 4.5 mm.

The lumen of the nozzle should be not less than 1.2 mm.

5.1.6 The Plunger and Piston

The plunger should be designed to be pushed by the thumb from the pushed button while the barrel was held by one hand from the finger grips. When the fiducial line of the piston coincides with the zero point of the graduation, the projection of the push button from the finger grips is preferable to be as follows:

- For syringes < 2 ml is 8 mm.

- For syringes 2 ml to < 5 ml is 9 mm.

- For syringes 5 ml or more, the projection is 12.5 mm.

- The plunger should not be easily detachable from the barrel.

- When the syringe is filled with water and held vertically, the plunger shall not move by its own mass.

5.1.7 Performance

5.1.7.1 Dead space

The volume of liquid remained in the barrel and nozzle after fully insertion of the piston conceding with the zero point. The requirements are demonstrated in table (5-2).

Procedure:

- Weigh the empty syringe using a digital balance capable of determining a mass difference of 0.2 gm or less and of accuracy of 7 mg.

- Fill the syringe with distilled water to its nominal capacity, expel the air bubbles to ensure that the level of water coincides with the end of the nozzle lumen.

- Expel the water by fully depressing the plunger and dry the outer surface of the syringe.

- Re-weigh the syringe.

- As the density of water is 1gm/cm^3, the difference in mass represents the dead space.

- The dead space is expressed in millilitre for specific syringe nominal capacity.

Table (5-2) Dead space & forces for leakage testing

Capacity v ml	Dead space ml	Forces for leakage	
		Side force ±5% N	Axial pressure ±5% guage
V<2	0.07	0.25	300
2< v < 5	0.07	1	300
5< v < 10	0.075	2	300
10< v < 20	0.1	3	300
20< v < 30	0.15	3	200
30< v < 50	0.17	3	200
50 > v	0.2	3	200

5.1.7.2 Air and liquid leakage past the piston-Aspiration

There shall be no leakage of air or water past the piston or seal. Table (5-2) shows the forces for leakage testing.

There are three results required from the test:

1- There should be no air or liquid past the piston or seal.

2- There should be no fall in pressure less than 60 ± 5.

3- The piston will be checked if it is leaking from the plunger or not.

Figure (5-2) The diagram and picture of the apparatus.

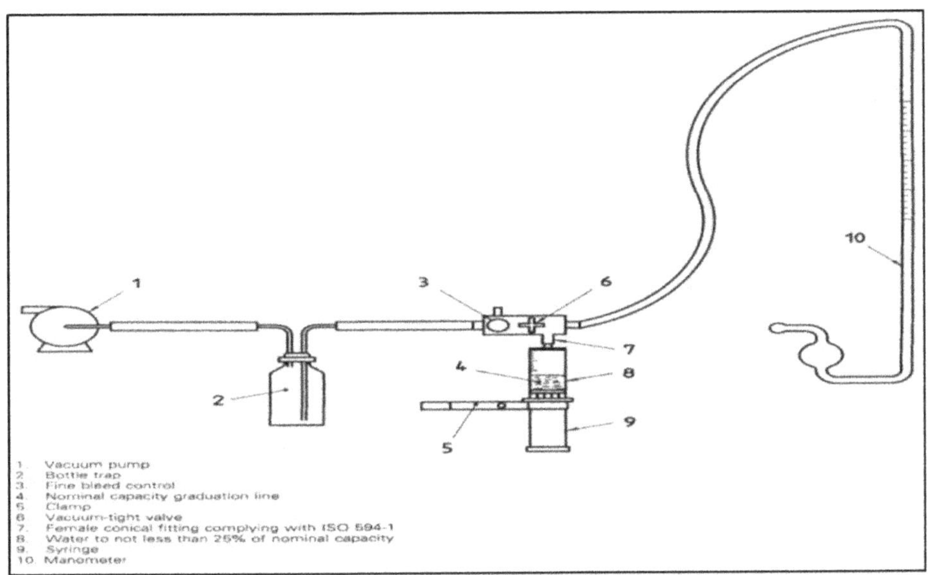

Figure (5-3) ISO 7886-1 USP 132/ USP 382: plunger glide force for syringe leakage Test Apparatus [Zwick Roell]

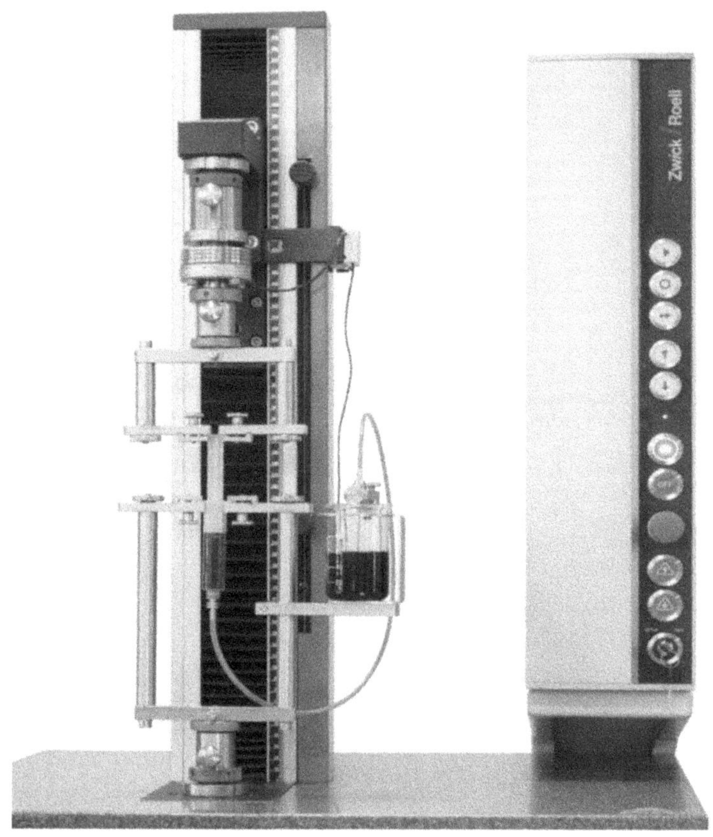

The syringe nozzle is connected to reference female conical hub and the syringe is filled to not less than 25% of its nominal capacity. Negative pressure is applied through the nozzle and the syringe inspected for leakage past the piston and if the piston is detached from the plunger.

Procedure:

1- Draw into the syringe a volume of water not less than 25% of its nominal capacity. The water was freshly boiled and cooled to 20 ± 5 °C.

2- Withdraw the plunger, through the nozzle opening, to the fiducial line at the nominal capacity graduation line and clamp the plunger on this position.

3- Connect the syringe nozzle to the reference female conical fitting.

4- Connect the apparatus and switch on the pump with the air bleed control open.

5- Adjust the bleed control so that the pressure is reduced gradually until the manometer reading is 88 kpa below the atmospheric pressure.

6- Examine the syringe leakage of air past the piston or seal.

7- Isolate the syringe and the manometer assembly and observe the manometer reading at 60 ± 5 and record any fall in the reading.

8- Examine the piston if it is detached from the plunger.

5.1.7.3 Testing liquid leakage at syringe piston under compression

The syringe is filled with water, the nozzle is sealed and the plunger is arranged at the worst position. Force is applied in an unfavorable direction to induce leakage. Apparatus ZYT-01 ISO 7886 liquid leakage tester at syringe plunger stopper under compression is used. It applies positive pressure and test the tightness of all syringe body, figure (3-3).

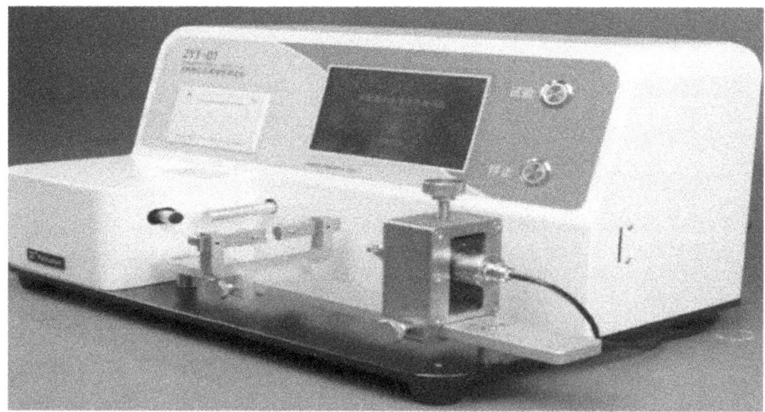

Figure (5-4) Leakage tester Z Pubtester instrument-China

5.1.7.4 Forces required for operating the plunger

An apparatus as in figure (3-4) is used to move the plunger to aspirate and expel water while the forces exerted during plunger movement is recorded.

Figure (5-5, 6) Apparatus for determining the forces to operate the plunger of syringe-ISO 7886-1 Annex G

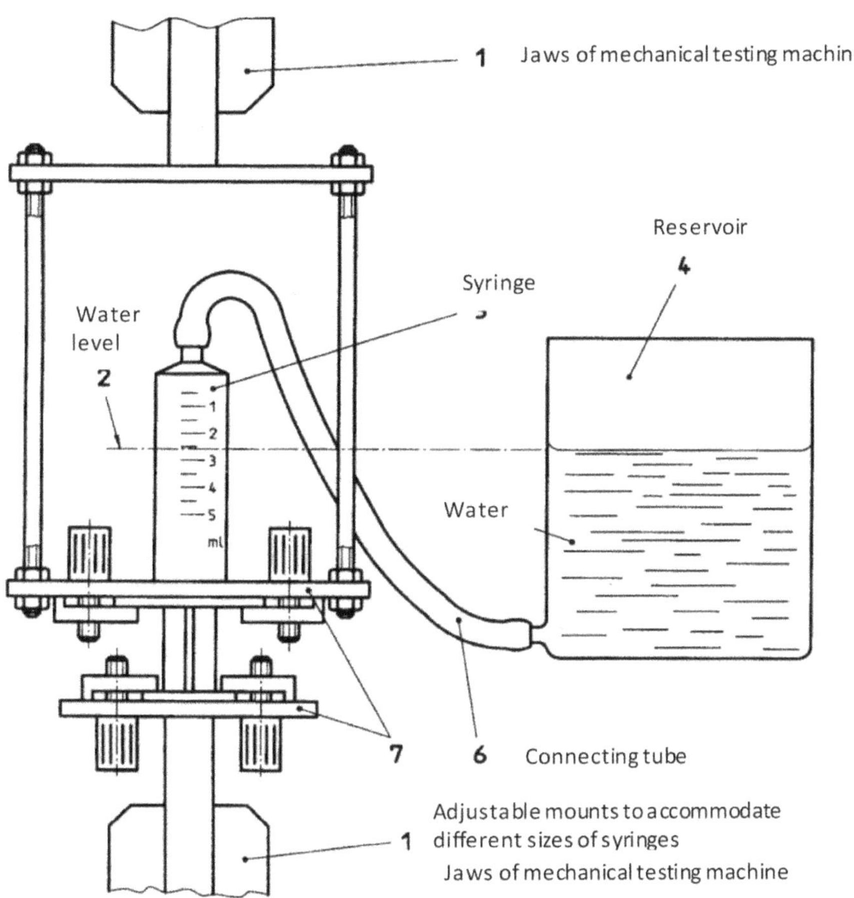

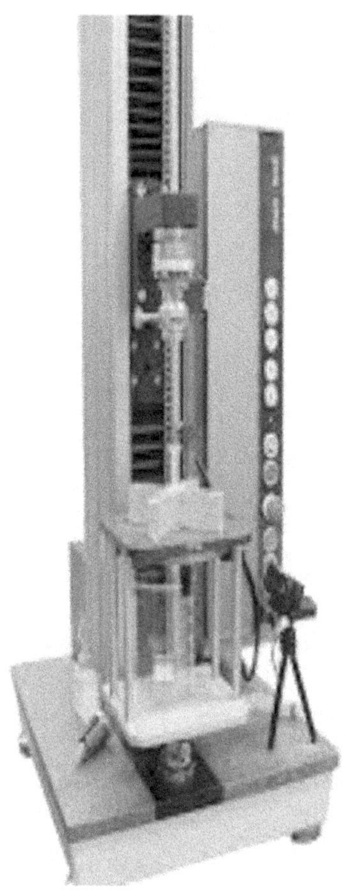

Procedure:

1- Mount the syringe to be tested, move the syringe plunger to full capacity and return it back to the zero-graduation line.

2- Connect the nozzle to the tube of the reservoir, maintain the reservoir water at 23 ±2 °C. then free the tube from any air bubbles.

3- Maintain the water level in the reservoir and in the syringe at the same level as in the diagram.

4- Set the recorder at zero point and set the machine to apply compression and tensile strengths without re-setting.

5- Start testing so that the plunger withdrawn at a speed of 100 ±5 mm/min until it reached the nominal full capacity line of graduation. Thus, water will be withdrawn from the reservoir to the syringe.

6- Stop the apparatus and set the pressure at zero and wait for 30 seconds.

7- Reverse the machine and return the plunger to its original position, so that the expelling water from the syringe to the reservoir.

Record the following forces:

F_s: force in N required to initiate the movement of the plunger.

F_m: mean force in N during return of the plunger.

F_{max}: maximum force in N during return of the plunger.

F_{min}: minimum force in N during return of the plunger.

Table (5-3) The proposed forces required to operate the plunger

Nominal capacity V	F_s N	F_m N	F_{max} N	F_{min} N
V< 2 ml	10	5	2 x F_m or F_m + 1.5 N whichever is lower.	0.5 x F_m or F_m – 1.5 N Whichever is higher
2 £ v <50 ml	25	10		
50 £ v ml	30	15		

5.2 Requirements and Tests for Needle

The European Committee for Standardization EN: ISO 7864 on hypodermic needle having 6% luer conical fitting and sizes from 0.3mm outer diameter to 1.2 mm.

Tests should be applied to sterilized product and using statistical measures of accuracy and precision regarding the calibration and repeatability and reproducibility for testing of gauge. The needle surface should be from particle or extraneous matter when inspected by normal vision without magnification on illumination of 300-700 lx. On magnification of 2.5 the hub shall appear free from particles or extraneous matter.

5.2.1 Packaging and Labelling

Primary container:

Contains description of content, metric size, sterile, lot number, and trade name.

Secondary container:

Contains metric size, angle of bevel, wall thickness, sterile, for single use, lot number, warning to check the integrity.

5.2.2 limit for Acidity, Alkalinity and Extractable Metal

A-Preparation of the test extract S,

Immerse 25 needles in 250 ml deionized or distilled water in a suitable borosilicate glass container. Ensure complete immersion of the needles in water and maintain the temperature at 37 ± 3 °C for 60 ± 2 minutes. Remove the needles and ensure no water is on the surface of the needles.

All water is in the container. Perform a control fluid without immersion of needles.

B-Limit for the pH

The pH of the extract shall be within 1 unit that of the control fluid.

C-Limit for the extractable metal

The extract contains not more than 5 mg/ litre of lead, tin, zinc and iron. Cadmium is lower than 0.1 mg/litre (tested by atomic absorption figure (5-7).

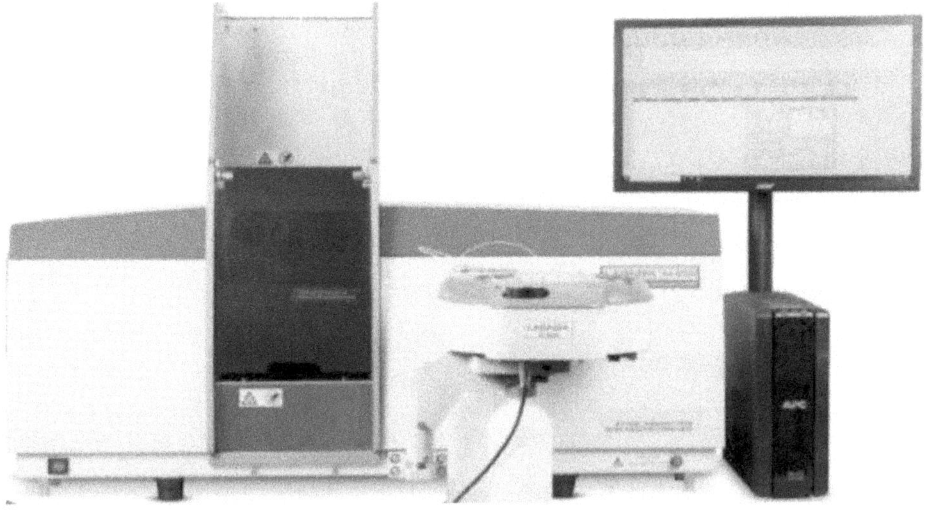

Atomic absorption spectrophotometer *Perkins Elimar*

5.2.3 Morphology and Dimensions

5.2.3.1 morphology of the needle

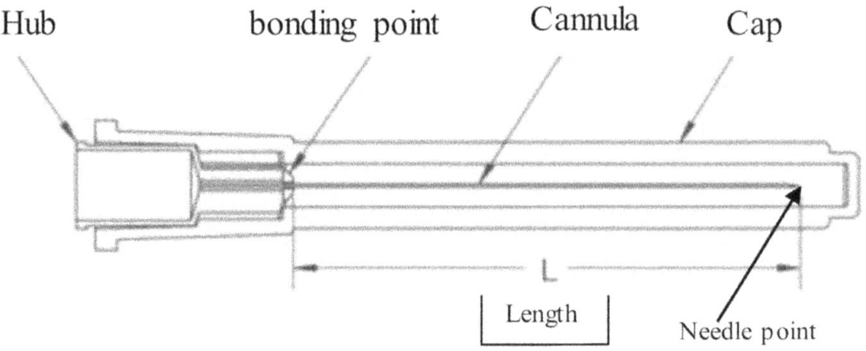

Figure (5-8) demonstrates different parts of the needle.

5.2.3.2 Needle tube

The needle tube or cannula should be straight, regular shape and free from defects. It may be tubular or tapered.

a. Tubular designation

Tubular needle may be expressed in gauge and the length is in mm, the wall thickness may be expressed as regular wall, thin wall, extra-thin or ultra-thin wall. E.g. 0.8 mm x 40 mm TW.

b. Tapered needle designation:

The outer diameter at the hub end is greater than that at the tip point. It is expressed as OD hub/ OD tip by length e.g: 0.23mm/0.255mm x 6 mm TW

c-Length

The actual length of the needle shall equal the nominal length within the tolerance described in table (3-4)

Table (5-4) tolerance for the length of the tube

Nominal length	Upper tolerance	Lower tolerance
< 25 mm	+1 mm	2 mm
25 – 39 mm	+ 1.5 mm	2.5 mm
40 mm	0	4 mm
>40 mm	+ 1.5 mm	2.5

d-Lubrication

The lubricant should not be visible on visual inspection neither in droplets nor in particle on the surface of the needle. Polydimethyle siloxane is used in quantity not exceeding 0.25 mg per square centimeter of the surface area of the needle.

5.2.3.3 The needle point

On 2.5 magnification, the needle sharpness bevel angle tip shall appear free from feather edges, burrs and hooks. The bevel angle is 11°±2, but if shorter bevel the angle may be 17°±2.

The angle can be determined by needle sharpness tester and through the force required for penetration. Figure (3-9) shows the details of tip point parts.

Figure (5-9) Needle tip point-Wikipidia.org

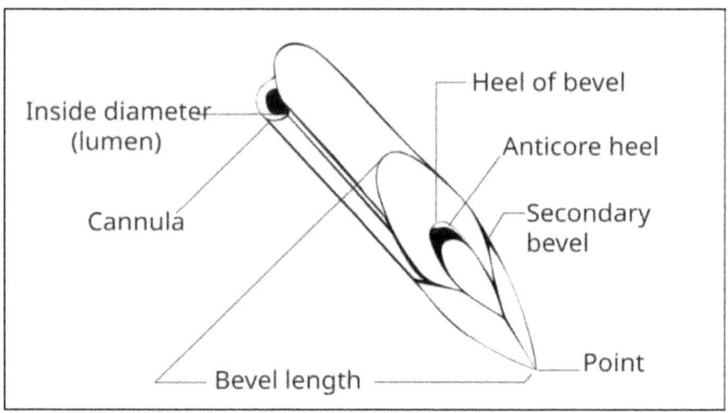

Figure (5-10) Needle sharpness Tester CIA Medical-USA

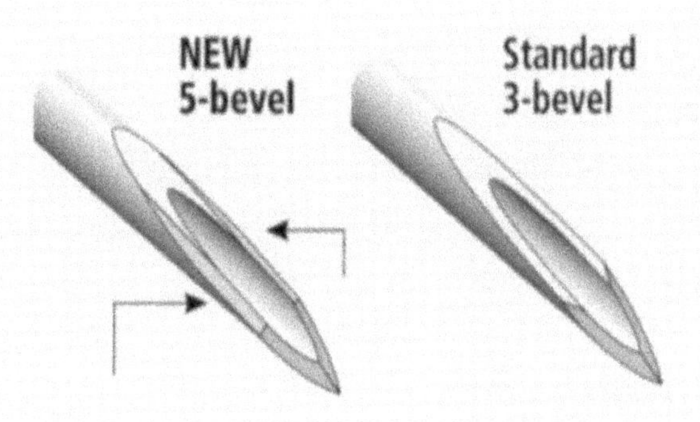

CIA medical company US innovate 5-bevel needle which is more comfortable than 3-bevel figure (5-10).

5.2.4 Patency of Lumen

To carry out the test for determining the measurement and patency of the needle lumen, a stainless steal stylet of relative diameter to the nominal diameter in table (3-5) is to be passed through the needle.

Table (5-5) Determination of the lumen patency

Outer diameter	Stylet diameter mm		
of needle mm	Normal walled	Thin walled	Thick walled
0.3	0.11	0.13	-
0.33	0.11	0.15	-
0.36	0.11	0.15	-
0.4	0.15	0.19	-
0.45	0.18	0.23	-
0.5	0.18	0.23	-
0.55	0.22	0.27	-
0.6	0.25	0.29	0.3
0.7	0.3	0.35	0.37
0.8	0.4	0.42	0.44
0.9	0.48	0.49	0.5
1.1	0.58	0.6	0.68
1.2	0.7	0.73	0.83

1. The rate of flow of water through the needle under hydrostatic pressure of $1 \times 10^5 Pa$, shall not be less than 80% of a needle of equivalent outer diameter and length having minimum inner diameter in accordance with ISO 9626 when tested under the same pressure.

5.2.5 Flow Rate Through the Needle Test

Flow of water through the needle requires the use of qualified calibrated flowmeter the diagram of the process is demonstrated on figure (3-11).

Figure (5-11) Determination of flow rate of needle

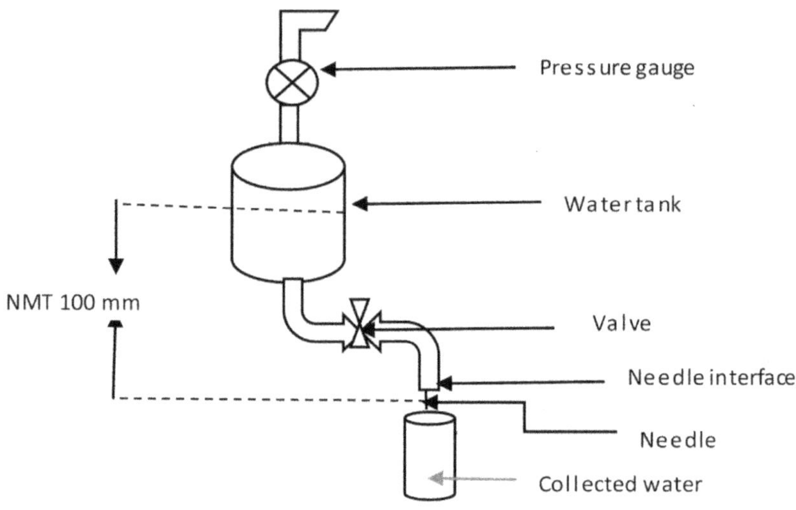

1. Fill the water tank with water at 23 ±2 °C.

2. Connect the tested needle in the test fixture that is connected to the tank.

3. Use pressure 1.1 bar for needles of o.6 mm OD and 0.11 bar for needles greater than 0.6 mm OD.

4. Water flow through the needle for 15 seconds and the reflux is collected.

5. Repeat the test for 20 samples from 3 batches.

6. Calculate the flow rate in milliliter per minute.

5.2.6 Bond Strength Between Hub and Needle Tube

The bond shall not be broken by minimum forces mentioned in table (3-6) when applied as pull or push directions.

Nominal outer diameter of needle	Minimum force in Newton
0.3 to 0.5 mm	22 N
0.55 to 0.6 mm	34 N
0.7 mm	40 N
0.8 mm	44 N
0.9 mm	54 N
1.1 mm	69 N
1.2 mm	69 N

<u>Apparatus: Universal Tensile Strength</u> figure (5-12)

- Load cell of max 500 N

- Test speed 50 mm/ minute.

1- the needle is vertically positioned on the apparatus.

2- grip the needle avoiding slipping.

3- set the load cell to zero, the load is zero.

4- apply test speed at 50 mm/ minute.

5- start and record the maximum force to remove the needle from the hub or the needle or hub is broken.

6- maximum load (N) is the bonding force.

Figure (5-12A) Electric Universal Tensile strength tester.
Ebay.com from Szsosowin-China

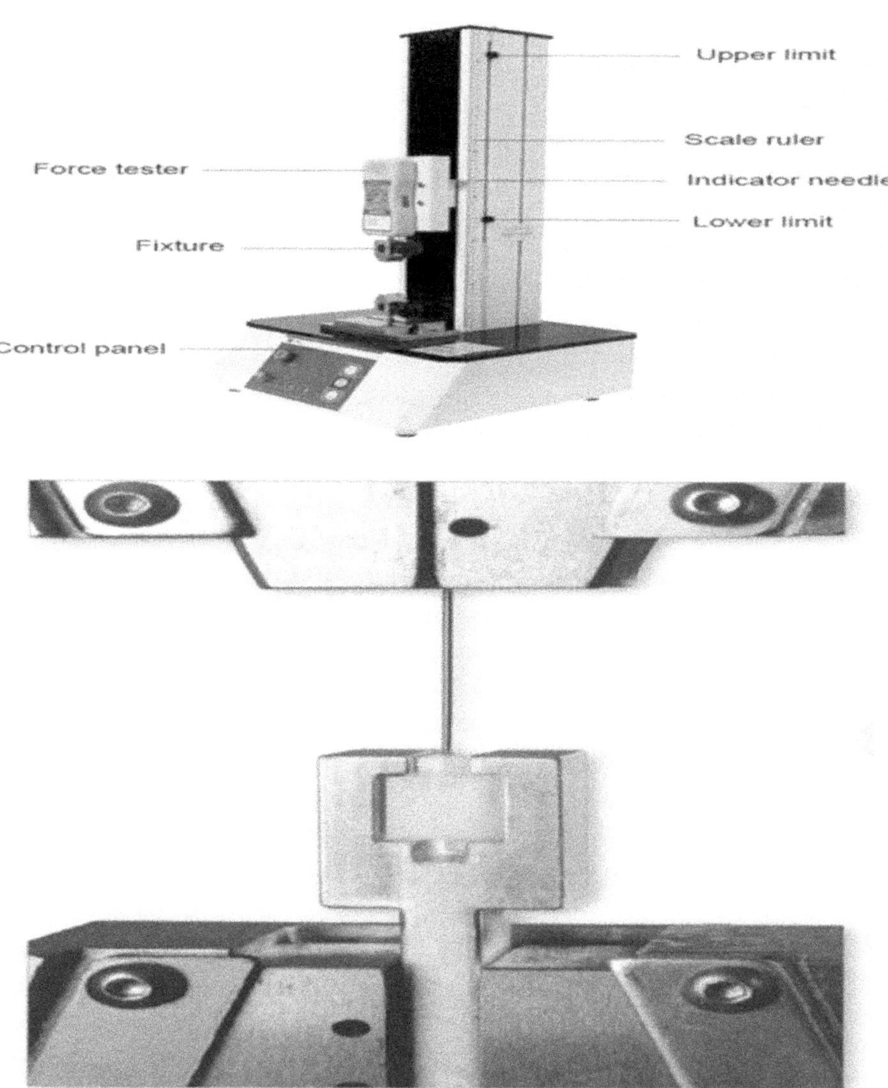

Figure (5-12 B) Pulling the needle.

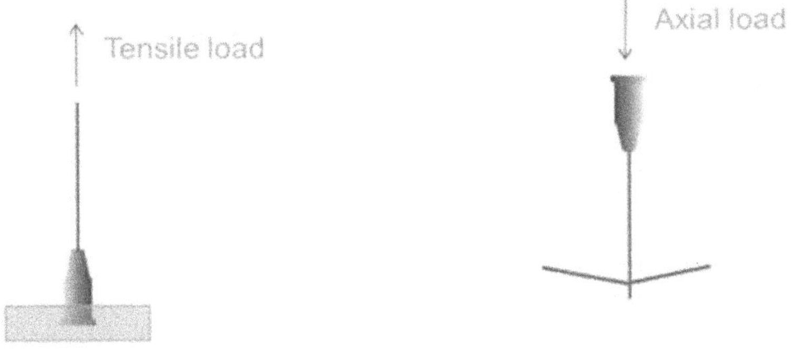

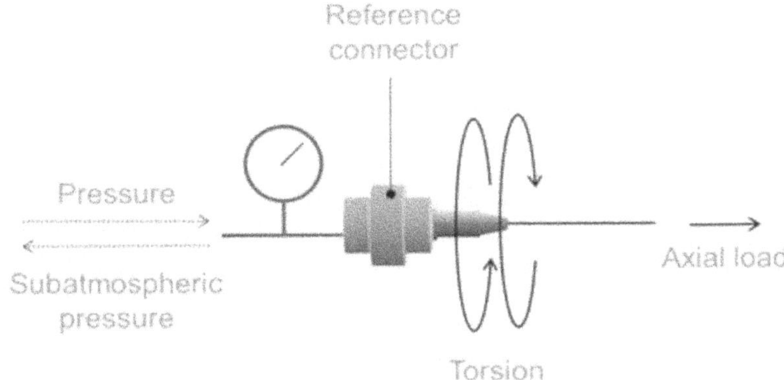

Figure (5-13) Direction of forces

5.2.7 Fragmentation Test

The test is informative as defined by IOS standard 7864 and the principle of which is that the penetration of the needle in the rubber will result in fragments which will be a defect in the finishing of the needle top point. So, standard rubber should be used and standard reference needle is used for comparing the results. The reference and test needles are let to penetrate a standard rubber of vial containing distilled water, then the contents of the vials are filtered and fragments are counted and compared.

Procedure: (ISO standards 8764-1)

1- fill a vail to 50% of its nominal capacity with distilled water.

2- place the standard rubber closure on the vial and grip by aluminum cap and inspect for the presence of fragments and reject any vial with fragments.

3- fill 10 ml syringe with water and fix to it the reference needle.

4- hold the vial vertically and also the syringe and pierce the closure as in figure (3-14).

5- inject 2 ml of water into the vial, withdraw the needle from the vial, remove the needle from the syringe and replace it by fresh reference needle.

6- repeat steps 4 and 5 for a total of 5 penetrations choosing different areas.

7- repeat steps 3, 4, 5, 6 on 5 vials (25 reference needles and 25 penetrations).

8- remove the closure, filter using a filter paper size 0.5 mm.

9- Inspect by normal vision without magnification, the distance between the eye and filter paper is 250 ±5 mm.

10- repeat steps 3, 4, 5, 6, 7, 8 using 25 needles to be tested.

Record and compare the results.

Figure (5-14) Fragmentation Testing

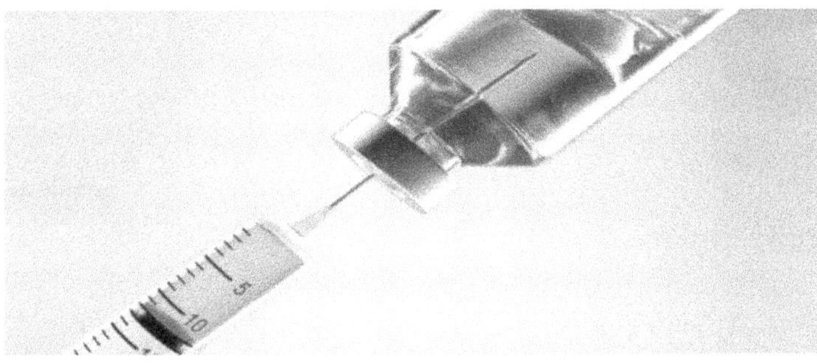

5.2.8 Measuring the Penetration Force and Drag Force

The penetration force which occur when the needle pierce the skin. This directly related to the pain felt by the patient. The smaller the penetration force, the lesser pain. A specific silicon skin as substrate is used to insert a needle at specific speed. The force of insertion is recorded as a function of penetration depth using a load cell. Measuring the initial penetration force and the force that keeping the needle drag or move through the substrate.

A typical test speed is 100 mm/minute.

The substrate

- normal rubber having hardness 40 ± 5 Shore A and thickness 1 ± 0.1 mm.

- Polyurethane of hardness 85 ± 10 Shore A and of thickness 0.4 ± 0.05 mm.

- Silicon rubber of hardness 50 ± 5 Shore A and of thickness 0.5 ± 0.05.

- Polyethylene HDPE of thickness 50 ± 5 mm.

The substrate is fixed between two plates. The plate having a penetration void of diameter of 10 mm as in figure (3-15 a-c).

The penetration depth is 80% of the needle length.

Measure the maximum force required to penetrate the substrate, this is the penetration force.

Measure the average force required to reach 80% of the needle length, this the drag force.

Figure (5-15a) diagrammatic presentation for penetration

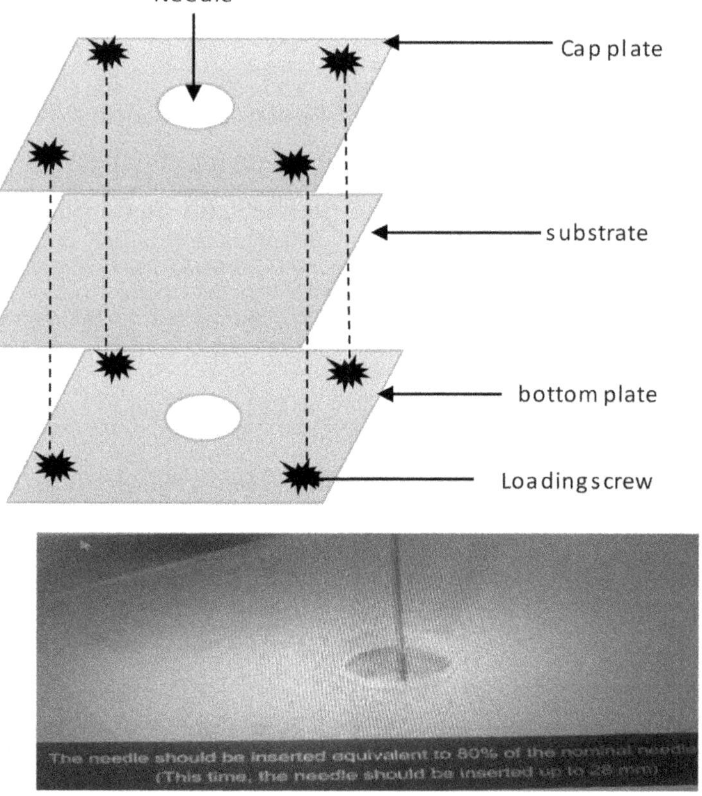

Figure (5-15b) Penetration force and drag force tester-
Eqvimech – m.indiamart.com, Thane

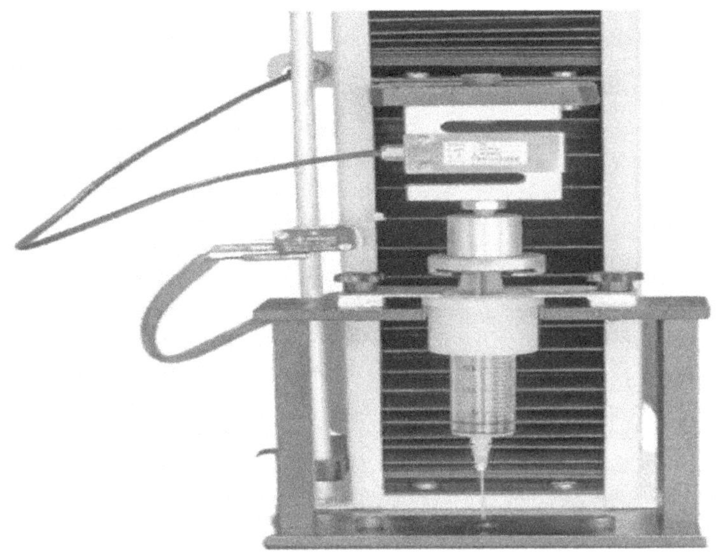

Figure (5—15c) Graphical determination of forces
(by software). Penetration force drag force

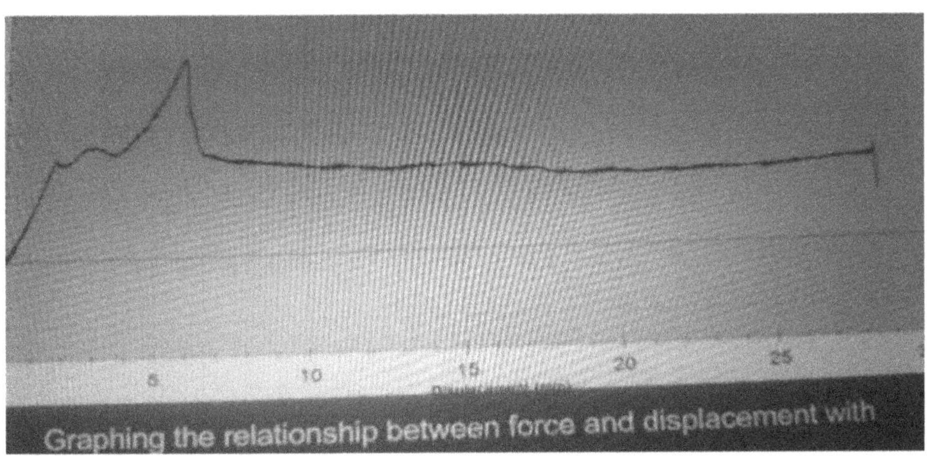

5.2.9 Stiffness Test

A- The break resistance of needle is determined according to the ISO Standard 9626 (Annex C) using two point flexure test. The needle is held on one side and the other side is bent at a definite angle as in figure (3-16).

Figure (5-16) bending of needle. *ZwickRoell*

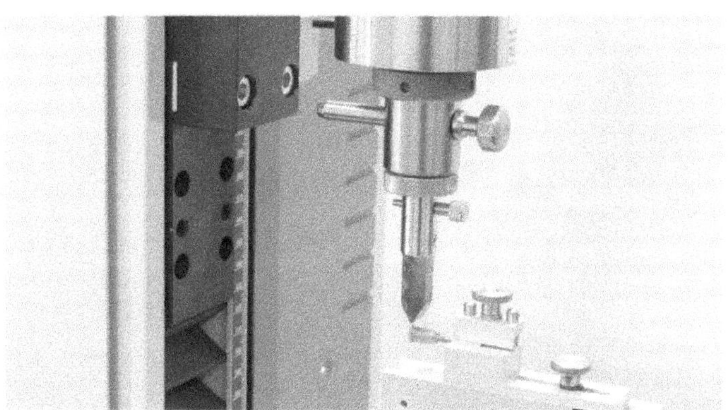

B- The Standard DIN EN 9626 (Annex B) defines the stiffness test as 3-point flexure. Apply specified force to the centre of the specified span of needle supported and fixed at both ends and measure the deflection value and load on the needle tube. The applied bending force is measured by rigidity tester by special sensor that measure and record the rigidity of the needle tube at the point of application.

5.3 Chemical Tests for the Complete Syringe

The pharmacopoeia defines the most important tests for the disposable syringe.

1- quantification of silicon oil; the lubricant.

2- quantification of residual Ethylene Oxide gas.

Figure (5-17) Three-point stiffness tester, Instron.com-US

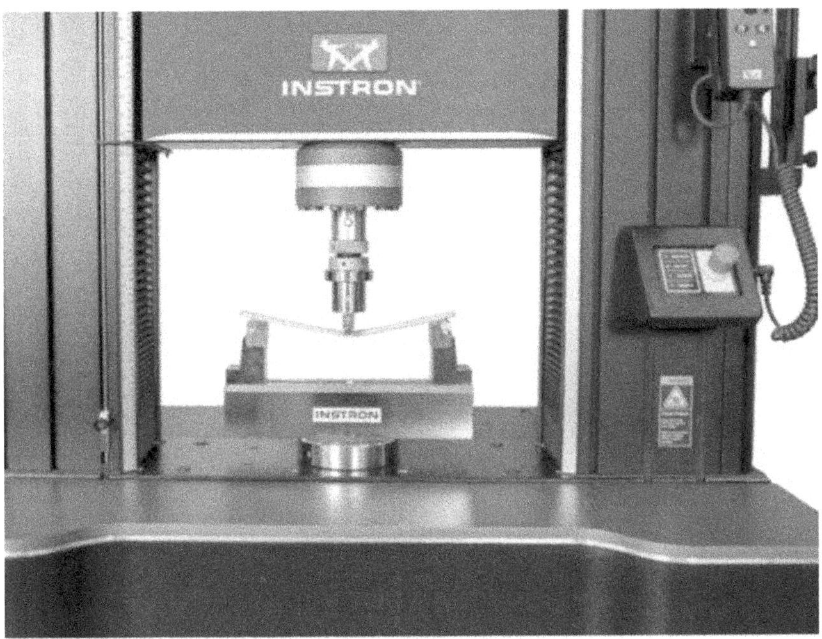

5.3.1 Test and Requirements for Silicon Oil

The Ph.Eur. method (3.2.8), Appendix XIX G. Sterile Single-Use Plastic syringe describes the method for determination of silicon oil in the plastic syringe as follows:

1- Calculate the internal surface area of the syringe using the equation $2\sqrt{V}.\pi.h$

   Where V: is the nominal volume of the syringe in cm^2.

   h: is the height of the graduation in cm.

2- Take sufficient number of syringes to give surface area from 100-200 cm^2.

3- Aspirate into each syringe methyl chloride to half its nominal volume and air to the other half.

4- Rinse the internal surface area with solvent by inverting the syringe 10 times in succession with the needle closed by plastic inert to methyl chloride and fixed by finger.

5- Expel the extract into tared dish and repeat the operation.

6- Evaporate the combined extract to dryness on a water bath.

7- Dry at $100 - 105$ °C for 1 hour.

→ The residue weight not more than 0.25 mg/ cm^2 of the surface area.

8- Examine the residue by Infrared absorption Spectrometer.

→ It shows absorption bands typical to silicon oil at 805 cm^{-1}, 1020 cm^{-1}, 1095 cm^{-1}, 1260 cm^{-1}, and 2960 cm^{-1}.

Figure (5-18) Infrared Spectrometer

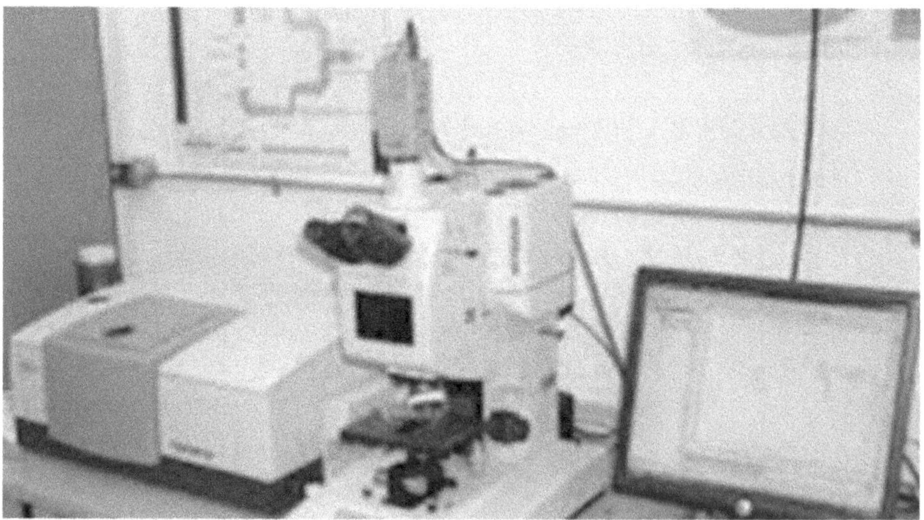

5.3.2 Test and Requirements for Residual Ethylene Oxide Gas

According to Ph.Eur. Method 2.2.28, the test for residual ethylene oxide is carried out by Gas Chromatography.

Chromatographic conditions:

- Column made of stainless steel having 1.m length and 6.4 mm internal diameter packed with salinized diatomaceous earth for gas chromatography R impregnated with macrogol 1500 R (3 gm/ 10 gm).

- Helium gas for chromatography as carrier gas.

- Flow rate 20 ml/min.

- Detector: flame ionization detector.

Temperature:

- Temperature of the column: 40 °C.

- Temperature of the injector: 100°C.

- Temperature of the detector: 150°C.

Ethylene oxide solution:

- Preparation should be carried out in fume cabinet.

- In a 50 ml vial, place 50 ml dimethylacetamide R, stopper the vial securely a weigh to the nearest 0.1 mg.

- 50 ml PP or PE syringe, fill with ETO gas, leave for 3 minutes, empty the syringe and fill again with 50 ml ETO gas.

- Place the needle and reduce the volume of gas to 25 ml.

- Inject these 25 ml into the vial.

- Gently shake the content and avoid the contact to the needle.

- Weigh the vial again and record the increase in mass.

- The increase in mass is 45 mg – 60 mg is used to calculate the exact concentration of ETO in solution. It is about 1 gm/litre.

Calibration curve:

1- prepare 7 vials filled with 50 ml dimethylacetamide R. and in each vial place the respective ETO:

   0 ml, 0.02 ml, 0.05 ml, 0.1 ml, 0.5 ml, 1 ml and 2 ml.

2- stopper securely and place the vials in an oven at $70 \pm 1°C$ for 16 hours.

3- take 1 ml of the hot gas from each vial and inject into the column and draw the calibration curve; height of peak against mass of ETO, figure (3-19) will be obtained.

Figure 5-19: Calibration of ETO, gas chromatography.

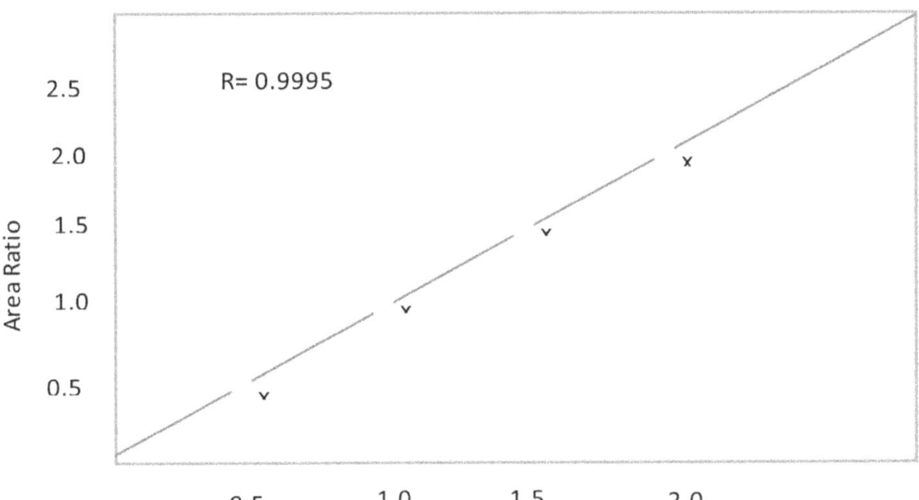

Test

1- weigh the syringe after removal of packaging.

2- Cut the syringe into pieces of maximum 1 cm dimensions and place in 250 ml – 500 ml vial containing 150 ml dimethylacetamide R.

3- Stopper securely and place in an oven at $70 \pm 1°C$ for 16 hours.

4- Remove 1ml of the hot gas and inject into the column, figure (3-20) will be obtain.

- From the calibration curve obtain the concentration corresponding to the peak height of the test.

Figure (5-20) Gas chromatography and ETO peak

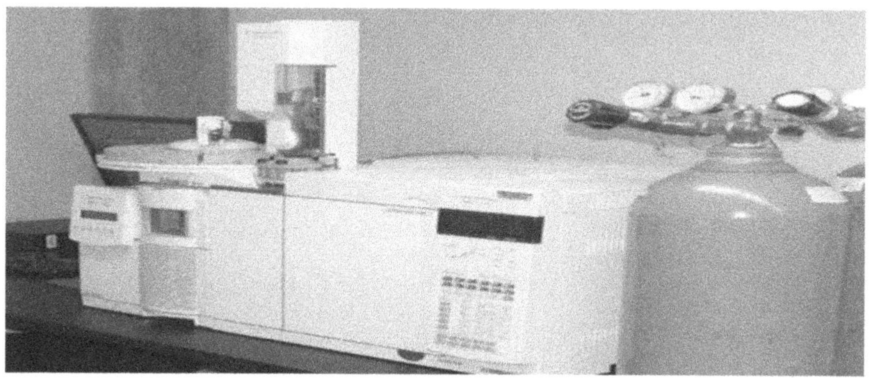

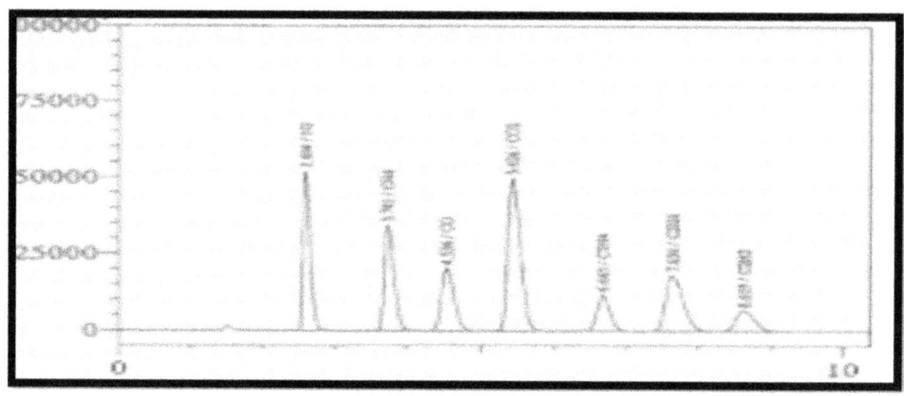

Ethylene Oxide residue should not be more than 10ppm.

5.4 Microbiological Requirements and Tests

The sterile single-use plastic syringe should be sterile and specifies pyrogen test for nominal volume more than 15 ml.

The microbiological tests should be carried out in a laminar flow cabinet to void extraneous contamination.

In all case the syringe shall be removed from the package aseptically and using aseptic techniques in all steps of the test.

5.4.1 Sterility Test

1- Aseptically, remove the package of the syringe.

2- Dismantle the syringe components.

3- Place each of the components in a container containing a sufficient amount of culture medium to cover the part completely.

4- Use both recommended media are as follows:

a. Fluid thioglycolate medium: for anerobic and aerobic bacteria incubated at 30-35°C.

b. Soya-bean casein digest medium.: for fungi and aerobic bacteria and incubated at 20-25°C for fungi.

→ Incubation period is 14 days.

There should be a negative and positive control, for the positive control use not more 100 cfu inoculation.

For thioglycolate medium use: *Clostridium sporogeneous, pseudomonas aeruginosa, staphylococcus aureus.*

For soya-bean casein digest medium use: *Aspergillus niger, Bacillus subtilis and Candida albicans.*

Incubate for 3 days in case of bacteria and 5 days for fungi.

5.4.2 Pyrogen Test

5.4.2.1 Rabbit pyrogen test

The Ph.Eur pyrogen test 2.6.8, Rabbit pyrogen test RPT

Syringes with a nominal volume equal to or greater than 15 mL comply with the test for pyrogens. Fill a minimum of three syringes to their nominal volume with a pyrogen-free 9 g/L solution of sodium chloride R and maintain at a temperature of 37 °C for 2 h. Combine the solutions aseptically in a pyrogen-free container and carry out the test immediately. Inject per kilogram of the rabbit's mass 10 mL of the solution into the marginal ear vein of rabbit as in figure (3-21).

The temperature was tested every 30 minutes, 40 minutes before injection up to three hours by a thermometer from rectum of the rabbit. Table (3-7) show the interpretation of results.

Figure (5-21) Injection of the rabbit

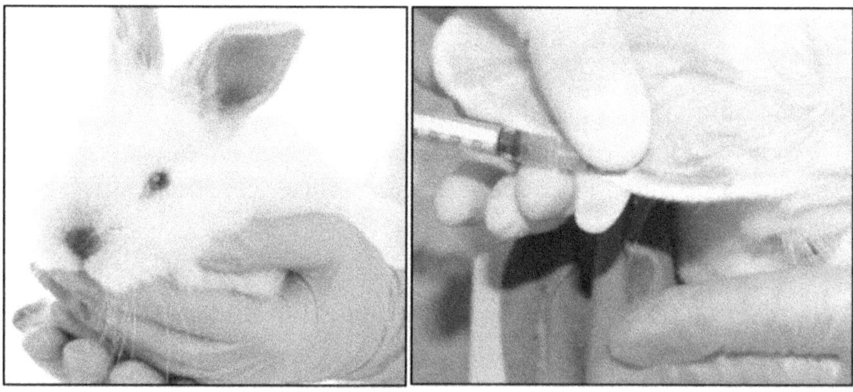

Table (5-7) interpretation of RPT results

No of rabbits	Passed if the summed response does not exceed:	Failed if the summed response is
3	1.15 °C	2.65°C
6	2.8°C	4.3°C
9	4.45°C	5.95°C
12	6.6°C	6.6°C

5.4.2.2 Monocyte-activation test Eur.Ph 2.6.30 MAT

Monocyte activation test was added to Eur Ph in 2009 as an alternative to RPT. This test is capable to detect endotoxin and non-endotoxin pyrogens.

In 28/06/2021 the Ph Eur announced the end of using the RPT.

Principle:

The human monocyte secretes pro-inflammatory cytokines such as interlukine-6 (IL-6) responding to the presence of endotoxin or pyrogen. This (IL-6) is linked to human fever reaction pathogenesis. These cytokines are quantitated using IL-6 ELISA assay. The solution to be tested is incubated with a source of human monocytic cell at $37\pm1°C$, 5% CO_2 in a humified air for a period sufficient to allow accumulation read-out, usually overnight (18 – 24) hours. The responses are compared to standard endotoxin or a reference lot of the preparation to be examined.

The apparatus used should be free from pyrogen usually glassware is heated to 250°C for 30 minutes. Plastic parts should be free from pyrogen.

Sources of monocytic cells:

1/ Whole blood.

2/ Peripheral blood mononuclear cells (pBMC) from a qualified donor.

The measured cytokine concentration is converted to endotoxin equivalent units per milliliter EU/ml using standard curve of lipopolysaccharide LPS. This conversion allows for quantitative assessment of endotoxin level in the product.

The Pelikine Human IL-6 Rapid ELISA kit allows detection of IL-6 cytokine in just 2 hours. Now it is included in all pyrocell MAT Rapid System Kit.

The Enzyme-Linked Immunosorbent Assay ELISA

The ELISA assay is a solid phase type of enzyme immunoassay to detect the presence of ligands usually protein in a liquid sample using antibodies directed against the ligand to be measured.

Antigens from the sample to be tested are attached to a surface. Then a matching antibody is applied over the surface so it can bind the antigen.

This antibody is linked to an enzyme and then any unbound bodies are removed. The substance containing the enzyme substrate is added. If there was any binding, there will be colour change.

Performing ELISA involves at least one antibody with specificity for a particular antigen.

The sample with a known amount of antigen is immobilized on the solid support usually polystyrene microtiter place (NUNC immune plate 96 well as figure 3-22) via adsorption or via capture by another antibody specific to the same antigen in a sandwich manner.

After the antigen is immobilized, the detection antibody is added forming a complex with the antigen. The detection antibody can be covalently linked to an enzyme or can be itself detected by a secondary antibody that is linked to an enzyme through bioconjugation. Between each step the plate is washed with a mild detergent solution to remove any protein or antibodies that are non-specifically bound. After the final wash step, the plate is developed by adding an enzymatic substrate to produce a visible signal (colour) which indicate the quantity of antigen in the sample.

Components of the kit:

1- crypto-preserved peripheral blood mononuclear cell (pBMO) preparation from human donation.

2- An optimized FBS-based culture medium supplement. The kit is validated with IL-6 ELISA.

   → The crypto-preserved pMAT cells are thawed and incubated with the test substance in a cell culture step for 18-24 hours. Then the cell culture supernatants are harvested and the IL-6 cytokine released by human monocytes is detected with human IL-6 ELISA assay measured in absorbance reader using reference endotoxin dilutions. The optical density OD values are finally converted to endotoxin equivalents EE/ ml.

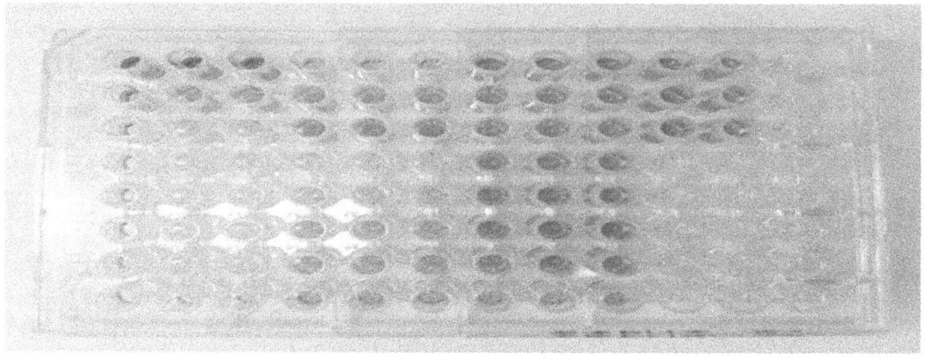

Figure 5-22A NUNC plate

Polystyrene plate of 96 well (microplates).

Process:

I. Step 1

Coat the ELISA 96 well cell culture plate with capture antibody, unbound antibody is removed and washed out. The capture antibody is that raised against the antigen to be detected.

II. Step 2

Cell supernatant is added, any antigen found in the sample will be captured by the antibody on the coat of the plate. Sample is applied in replicates and in varying concentrations to guarantee the levels of detection again any excess sample is washed out. (Figure 5-22)

(P.T.O)

Figure 5-22B: Application of sample for MAT test

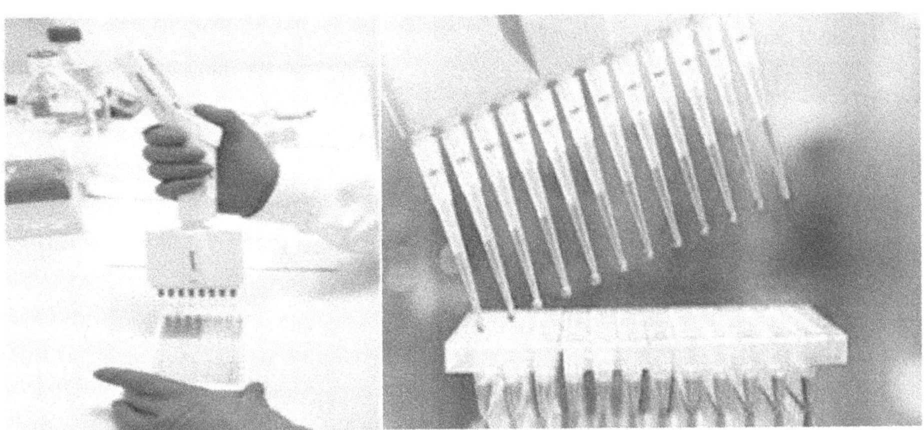

III. Step 3

Detection antibody is added. This antibody is labelled with an enzyme usually horse radish peroxidase or alkaline phosphatase. Detection antibody binds to the target antigen already bound to the plate.

IV. Step 4

The substrate is added to the plate. As ELISA is chromogenic, a reaction took place converting the substrate into a coloured product. The colour can be measured using plate reader. Figure 3-23 demonstrates the order of application of components.

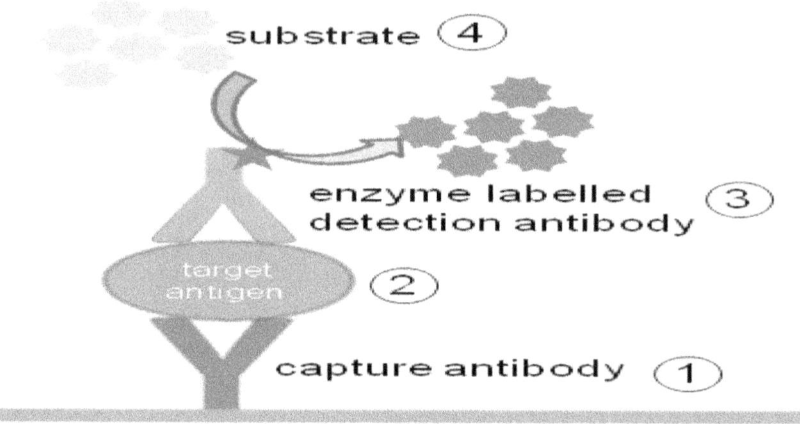

**Figure 5-23 Application of substrate and components.
[From the British Society for Immunology – London]**

V. Step 5

Read the results in microplate absorbance reader.

Determination of antigen concentration in the sample requires production of standard curve using antigen of known concentration, figure 3-24. The concentration of the antigen in the sample can then be calculated using the optical density OD.

Figure 5-24 standard antigen curve
(British Society for Immunology, London)

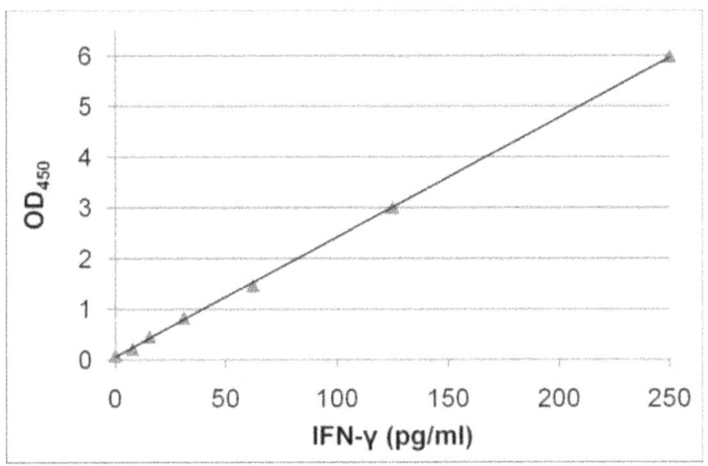

References

1. Asean Guidelines on Stability Study of drug product, May 2013, Indonesia.

2. Asean Validation Guidelines for pharmaceutical products, version 2, 2021.

3. Aulton M,2013, Aulton's Pharmaceutics, the design and manufacture of medicines, Churchill Livingstone,4th edition. PP 939-850.

4. British Society for Immunology, Enzymatic-Linked Immunosorbent Assay, ELISA, Bite-sized immunology.

5. Carlo P. Croce, Arthur Fischer and Thomas, Packaging materials science-4, The Theory and Practice of Industrial Pharmacy, Leon Lachman, Herbert and Kanic 1991, pp 711-731.

6. Carl Linter, Remington's pharmaceutical Sciences, 17th edition 1986, Pharmaceutical Press pp 1480.

7. China National Pharmaceutical Packaging Association, 2022, Study of Laminate film/bag for single-dose oral solution.

8. Donnel P and Bokser A,2005, Stability of Pharmaceutical Products,chapter 52, Remington 21, pp 1025-1036, 1034, published by Lippin-cott Williams and Wilkins.

9. EMA, European Medicine Agency, May 2000, Notes for Guidance on Specifications.

10. European Pharmacopoeia, Ph.Eur method 3.2.8, Ethylene Oxide Test, Appendix XIXG, Sterile single-use plastic syringes.

11. European Pharmacopoeia, Ph.Eur method 3.2.8, Silicone Oil Test, Appendix XIXG, Sterile single-use plastic syringes.

12. European Pharmacopoeia, Ph.Eur method 2.6.30 Monocyte-Activation Test MAT, 4299-4304.

13. Ezzet F, 2000, American Society for Microbiology, volume 44, No. 3 pp 297-700.

14. EMA, 2004, London, August 2004, ema CPMP/QWP/6142/03.

15. FDA sterility test, chapter 3.

16. FDA, Pharmaceutical Microbiology Manual, document 007.

17. FDA, Packaging and Labelling, container closure system for packaging human drugs and biologics. Guidance for Industry 1999, www.fda.gov

18. Gamil A, Effects of environmental conditions of Sudan on the Stability of Medicines, U of K, 2008.

19. Gamil A, Effects of transportation conditions across Sudan on the stability of medicines, Uof K 2009.

20. ICH, International Conference on Harmonization, 2004 Guidance for Industry Q1AR2, Q 6A, Q1E, Q1S, Q1F.

21. ICH, 2006, CPMP/ICH/42/02-June 2006.

22. Indian standards, 2022, Production Manual for sterile hypodermic syringes for single-use, Part1syringes for manual use, Bureau of Indian standards.

23. Indian Standards, 2002, sterile hypodermic needles for single use, Bureau of Indian Standards, New Delhi 110002, medical instruments and disposables sectional committee, MHD12, IS 10654:2002.

24. Indian Standards, 2002, sterile hypodermic syringes for single use, Bureau of Indian Standards, New Delhi 110002, medical instruments and disposables sectional committee, MHD12, IS 10258:2002.

25. Indian Mart, Pharmaceutical Packaging.

26. International Organization for Standardization ISO, 1993 (E), ISO 7886-1, Part 1, Syringes for manual use, Geneva 20, Switzerland.

27. International Standards Organization, ISO7886-1, 2017, 7866-2, 2020, 6866-3, 2020, 7886-4, 2018.

28. International organization for standardization,2016, ISO 7864, sterile hypodermic needle for single-use, requirements and testsfourth edition, 2016-08-01, www.iso.org

29. Kavita Bahmani and Hanyana, Quality Control for plastic container, slideshare, india.

30. Krisdiyanto M Eng et.al, the hypodermic syringe performance, Medicine, http://dx.doi.org/10./097/MD.0000000000031812.

31. Lucky S and Hij siti Mariam J, Aspects of quality assurance, WHO drug information, volume 18 no 2, 2004, pp 113-116.

32. Lonza Bioscience, Endotoxin and Pyrogen Testing, Monocyte-activation Testing MAT, https://bioscience.lonza.com

33. Martina Cambruzzi and Paul Macfarlane, 2021, Variation in yringe and needle dead space compared to the international organization for standardization ISO 7886-1:2018, Journal of Veterinary Anesthesia and Analgesia 48, http://doi.org/10.1016/j.vaa2021.01.008, PP 532-536.

34. Merck Millipore Sigma, Monocyte Activation Test,white papers, US and Canada.

35. NHS Pharmaceutical quality Assurance, 2013, Protocol for integrity testing of syringes, 2nd edition.

36. Princy Agarwal et.al Pharmaceutical Containers and Closure, http://inct.ac.in

37. Rabinow B and Roseman T, 2005, Plastic Packaging Material, Remington Pharmaceutical Sciences, chapter 54 pp 1025-1035. by Lippin-cott Wiliams Wilkins, 21th edition, 2005.

38. Royal Pharmaceutical Society of Great Birtain, 2014, packaging PP 132.

39. R. R. Evan, quality assurance for packaging in the pharmaceutical industry, Roussel Lab. Swidon, Witshire.

40. Savant D, 2021, Pharma pathway, 17th edition published by Nirali Parkashan.

190 • References

41. Sudaxshina Murdan, 2013, Packaging, Aulton's Pharmaceutical Sciences part 6, PP 811-825, Churchill Livingstone, Elsevier, Toronto, Canada.

42. The pharma Education website, https://www.thepharmaeducation.com

43. Thermo Sceintific, Nunc immune C8 star well. www.https://thermoscientific.com/oemdiagnostics

44. USP 30, 1/8/2007 for Windows by U.S pharmacopeia 12601 Twinbrook Pakway, Rockville,MD 20852 USA. Authentication No. 03-DXG15H1401. < 1191> < 1150>, <1151>, <1118>, < 1079>.

45. USP < 659 > Packaging and storage requirements, May 2017 (1-6)

46. USP < 660> containers – Glass pp 534, <71> sterility testing. <467> residual ethylene oxide, <232> Element Impurities Limits.

47. USP Extractable and Leachable, USP.org

48. USP.org <382> Elastomeric closure.

49. WHO 2012, Expert committee on specifications for pharmaceutical preparations, 46th report, technical report series 970.

50. WHO,2002, Guidelines on Packaging for pharmaceutical product, Technical report series No 902.

www.ingramcontent.com/pod-product-compliance
Lightning Source LLC
Chambersburg PA
CBHW042059150726
48005CB00032B/1187